# Mura Solwata Kosker

*'We Saltwater Women'*

# Mura Solwata Kosker

*'We Saltwater Women'*

ELLIE GAFFNEY AM

Routledge
Taylor & Francis Group
LONDON AND NEW YORK

Dedicated to 'Pumeri'
(Joseph Daniel McGinness OAM)
† 31 July 2003
Paperbark Man
Kungarakan Country, Northern Territory

# Foreword

Throughout her lifetime, Ellie Gaffney has been a strong advocate, both within Australia and internationally, of the interests and welfare of Torres Strait Islanders. She has been particularly committed to advancing the rights of Indigenous women. Her interests have spanned a wide spectrum of concerns.

As an administrator, Ellie Gaffney played a significant part in the development of hostel accommodation and primary health care for all Torres Strait Islanders. Ellie's work in establishing the Mura Kosker Sorority as a platform for change is widely recognised. At all times she has been an eloquent and determined presenter of the real situation of Torres Strait Islanders.

In recognition of her contribution to the Torres Strait and its people, Ellie was appointed a Member of the General Division of the Order of Australia (AM) in the Queen's Birthday Honours List (1990).

This memoir covers the period since the publication of her first book *Somebody Now* some 24 years ago. In doing so she shares with us and future generations her personal journey, a task she has undertaken at a time of failing health. It is a fitting reminder of the work and stature of a dedicated woman. Readers of this book will be inspired by Ellie Gaffney's efforts on behalf of Torres Strait Islanders and all Indigenous people.

*Aven Noah*

***Project development***

This project has been assisted by the Australian Government through the Australia Council, its arts funding and advisory body.

Australian Government

Australia Council for the Arts

First published 2007 by Goshawk Publishing

Published in 2016
by Routledge
2 Park Square, Milton Park, Abingdon, Oxon OX14 4RN
711 Third Avenue, New York, NY, 10017, USA

*Routledge is an imprint of the Taylor & Francis Group, an informa business*



---

**National Library of Australia Cataloguing-in-Publication data**

Gaffney, Ellie, 1932– .

Mura solwata kosker (we saltwater women).

ISBN 9780977574209.
ISBN 0 9775742 0 2.

1. Gaffney, Ellie, 1932– . 2. Torres Strait Islanders – Women – Biography. 3. Nurses – Queensland – Torres Strait Islands – Biography. 4. Indigenous women – Civil rights – Australia. 5. Torres Strait Islanders – Civil rights. 6. Torres Strait Islanders – Social conditions. I. Title.

920.00929912

---

ISBN 13: 9780977574209 (pbk)

# Contents

# Preface

I was born on 18 August 1932. I am a Torres Strait 'Solwata Woman', Wagadagum Tribe, of the Kadal and Dangal Totems. My father was Tomi Loban from Banda Neira, Indonesia. He was a pearl shell grader on Thursday Island. My mother was Geti Loban (*nee* Summers) from Mabuiag Island, Torres Strait.

This book I am writing is about the journey I wish to share with readers.

It has been 24 years since my first and only book *Somebody Now* was published and I have been approached by young Torres Strait women to document achievements since then.

My family also have encouraged me to try and accept this challenge because my medical problems restrict me, with time spent in hospital, and my physical and mental capacity of endurance. So, thank you Sylvia Tabuai for raising the issue.

My book is based on memory and reflection. There are many issues still facing Aboriginal and Torres Strait Islander people and I must put down my thoughts about them.

I leave behind in this book some ideas for the future so that others may learn from them.

*Ellie Gaffney* AM

# 1

# Joe McGinness: Dedication to a great man

Today (31st July 2003) is a sad day. It is when my friend and mentor, Joe McGinness, will be cremated. Joe died on NAIDOC (National Aborigines' and Islanders' Day Observance Committee) Day in Cairns.

Joseph Daniel 'Pumeri' McGinness was truly a remarkable and honourable Aboriginal man and we will miss him. Working for the rights of Aboriginal and Torres Strait people has been his whole life. He did this because he needed to and not for money, kickbacks or titles. He worked very hard with sincerity and hoped that his work would make a difference to our Aboriginal and Torres Strait peoples' endeavours.

He was an unselfish Aboriginal man who always turned his bitterness around into good and useful paths to advance the cause of Aboriginal and Torres Strait people. Joe told me whatever has been achieved in the way of reforms for Aborigines came about through the involvement and support of non-Aborigines, Church organisations and Federal trade unions which always showed compassion for the underprivileged. For the support given to him personally by the Waterside Worker's Federation, as he told me, he was forever grateful.

Joe was born in the country of the Kungarakan in the Northern Territory, known as the 'Paperbark people'. He was known as the son of Adyandabu. Uncle Joe, as we call him, because the kids call him that, left a legacy to every Aboriginal and Torres Strait person because of his involvement in the organisation FCAATSI (Federal Council for the Advancement of Aboriginals and Torres Strait Islanders). He became the first Indigenous President and held the position for seventeen years.

His other involvements were with the non-Aborigines, Church organisations and the Federal Trade Unions which gave him support and showed compassion for his fight for the under privileged. His legacy included Abstudy, Aboriginal Hostels, and better education, health and training programs to allow our Aboriginal and Torres Strait Islander people to develop and become educated and empower us to take control of our lives, destiny, politics, welfare, and housing and to be a human being with human rights, and not under the Australian Government's portfolio of Flora, Fauna, Fisheries and Aborigines in that order.

Uncle Joe's and FCAATSI's efforts brought about the 1967 Referendum to give us the rights that changed the lives of Aborigines and Torres Strait Islanders forever and which saw the Commonwealth Government legislate for funding to provide equal opportunity.

I honour those Torres Strait Islanders and Aboriginals who defied the government to remove the clauses from the Constitution which discriminated against Aboriginal and Torres Strait Islander people from their basic human rights. The Referendum, as we know now as history, succeeded, with a 91 per cent 'yes' vote to remove the exclusion clauses and gave us human rights. Remember in those days we never voted. It was the non-Indigenous voters who voted for us.

The FCAATSI grew out of the Victorian Aboriginal Advancement League. In 1956 the world was horrified by reports of bad health and sufferings of the Aboriginal people. A select committee was formed to investigate these matters.

In 1957 another select committee was formed and an Aboriginal, Doug Nicholls, was invited to be on the committee. When Doug Nicholls returned to Melbourne he called a public meeting and organised the showing of films of Aboriginals suffering in bad health.

FCAATSI became the national body with over 60 affiliated organisations from all over Australia. It played a major role in bringing about equal rights for Aboriginals and Torres Strait Islanders in wages, for example, like Wattie Creek, Land Rights, legislation to change laws providing equality with Europeans in education, housing, health and employment.

Because of FCAATSI we now enjoy freedom of speech and movements. We have better housing, education, health, hostels, jobs, ATSIC, TSRA, ICC and Legal Services. We were given a ministerial portfolio instead of being under the Minister for Flora, Fauna, Fisheries and Aboriginals.

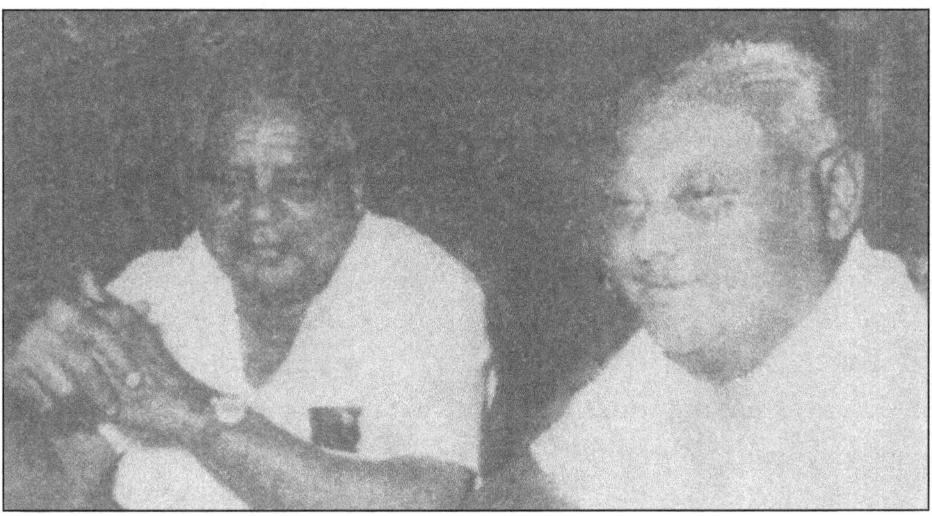

*Joe McGinness of West Cairns and Ted Loban of Thursday Island at Christine's Restaurant*

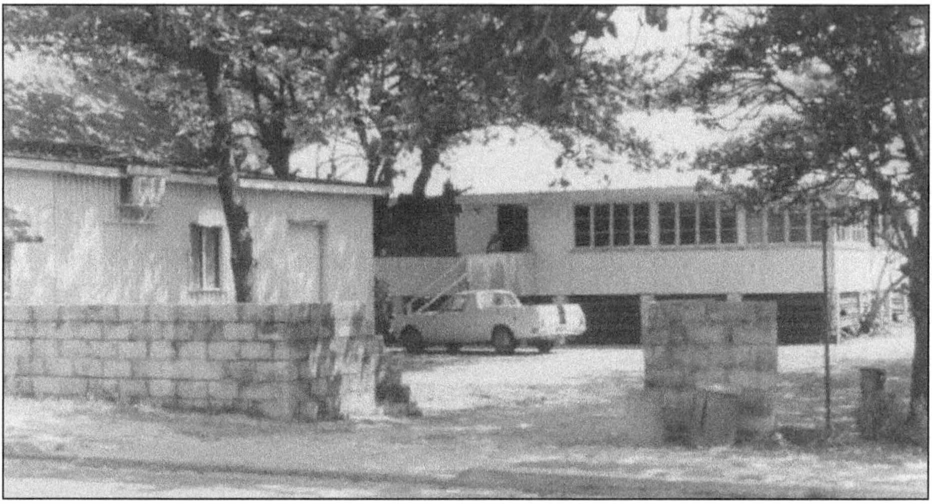

*Farquhar's house and store, Thursday Island, before demolition to build the Jummula Dubbins Aboriginal Hostel*

The Torres Strait Islands Aborigines in FCAATSI were Joe McGinness and Marjorie Wymarra. Joe lived on Thursday Island because his first and second wives were Torres Strait Islanders. Later in 1964 Joe co-opted TSI members, Ettie Pau, Elia Ware, Ted Loban and Jacob Abednego, and they became the freedom fighters.

Many families were living in humpies on the riverbanks and in shocking conditions throughout Australia and work was seasonal. When the season finished they became unemployed and homeless. Families could not afford to keep their children at school. If they were at school, a very few reached Grade 2, myself included. The health situation was extremely poor with a very high mortality rate, especially infant mortality.

Joe McGinness and Marjorie Wymarra saw that the Torres Strait situation was oppressed by the State Department of Native Affairs.

Joe McGinness went on to be the Regional Manager of North

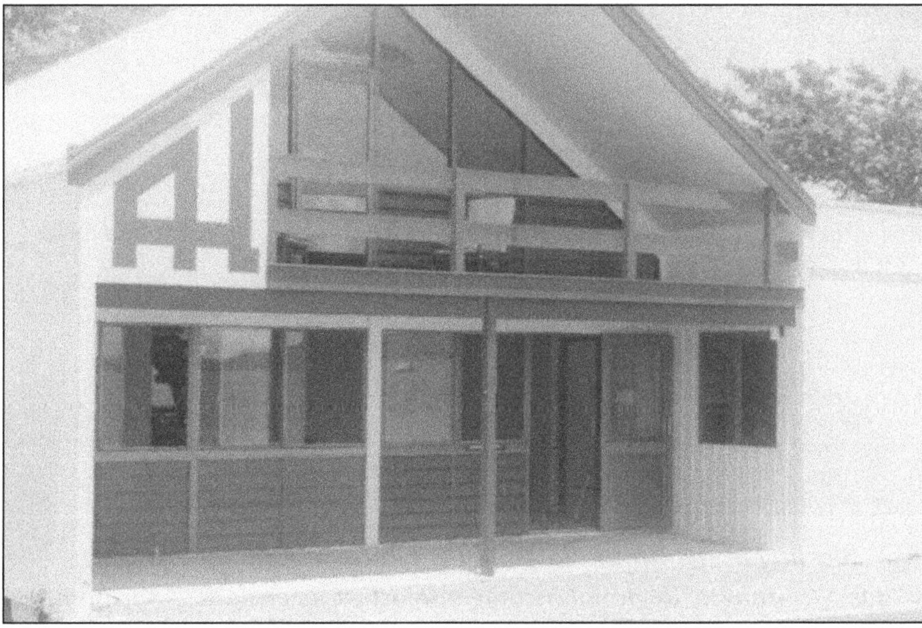

*Jummula Dubbins Aboriginal Hostel, the first on Thursday Island*

Queensland Aboriginal Hostels Ltd. He asked me to help him set up an Aboriginal Hostel on Thursday Island. Joe sought assistance from the QEH NACC (National Aboriginal Consultative Committee) member, Ted Loban, to purchase the Applied Ecology property which was originally the Farquhar's home and store on the waterfront.

This property was set up initially as the first hostel while Aboriginal Hostels Ltd was planning to refurbish and enlarge the accommodation. When Joe retired from active work and was replaced by Evelyn Scott, between them they employed me as the Hostel Manager with approval from the central AHL office in Canberra.

Uncle Joe based the needs of the underprivileged on his own life experience when he was put in the Kahlin Compound with his mother and the harsh times he endured there with other Compound

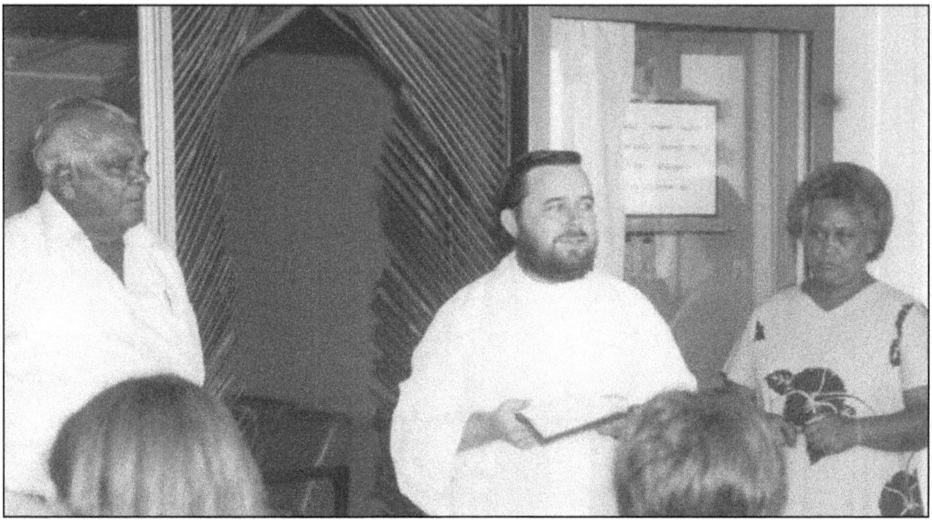

*Blessing of the Jummula Dubbins Hostel at Official Opening: Joe McGinness, Regional Manager, North Queensland Aboriginal Hostels Ltd (L), Fr Gordon Barnier, and Ellie Gaffney (R)*

kids. He never, never lost the will to improve his life and not let his spirit be broken.

What a remarkable journey for this Paperbark Man, from Compound kid to Dr Joseph Daniel McGinness, OAM.

He once said, 'As one of the Compound waifs there was no such thing as regular food or formal schooling for me or anything else for that matter.' Well, Uncle Joe, your lifetime work has filled many tummies with food, and privileged us with education so that we can take on the other things and do the things you fought for. *Kaima Eso* (big thank you). I am honoured and privileged to have known and worked with you.

2

# Social welfare

I worked for Hostels for three years during the development of the first Jummula Dubbins Hostel. During that time Joe McGinness and Evelyn Scott were concerned about the lack of social benefits for Torres Strait Islanders, similar to the benefits received by Indigenous people on the mainland.

The Islanders' social benefits were sent direct to the Department of Family Services and used as they saw fit. At an area advisory committee public meeting (the 'ICC' then), Evelyn Scott and Ted Loban raised this on the agenda, directing it at the Department of Social Security representative attending the meeting, who responded with an offer that if they could find someone to act as an agent and collect statistics, as well as to convince the Department in twelve months there was a need to establish an office for the Commonwealth Employment Service and the Department of Social Security, he would make it happen.

Evelyn and Ted accepted this offer and promptly nominated the Hostel's office for the service venue and the Manager, which was me. Words cannot express how dumbfounded I was. However, working with the Manager of the Department of Social Security, I developed a strategy to co-opt one island from each island group: Badu from the near western islands, Darnley from the eastern islands, Yorke from the central group, and Saibai from the top western group.

I contacted the Island Community Chairmen about the strategy

DEPARTMENT OF SOCIAL SECURITY

# AGENT APPOINTED

People needing Social Security information in the Thursday Island area now have a local person they can approach.

Mrs Ellie Gaffney has been appointed as an Agent for the Department of Social Security under a pilot scheme which will operate for 12 months. Mrs Gaffney can be contacted at Victoria Pde, Thursday Island. Her telephone number is Thursday Island 241.

Mrs Gaffney will work closely with the Manager of the Cairns office of the Department to —

- provide information about Social Security pensions, benefits and allowances;
- assist people in their general dealings with the Department;
- hold stock of departmental forms and leaflets;
- receive applications for assistance and other forms, such as the continuation for unemployment benefit.

Mrs Gaffney will not be able to provide highly technical information or make decisions. These matters are the responsibility of the staff of the Cairns office of the Department.

Mrs Gaffney will treat information given to her as confidential to her and the staff of the Cairns office of the Department.

The Department of Social Security is concerned to assist people who live outside those large centres which have Social Security offices. It is, therefore, appointing Agents such as Mrs Gaffney in 10 Queensland areas to test the value of this type of arrangement.

*Newspaper clip announcing appointment of the author as Agent for the Department of Social Security on Thursday Island, 1983*

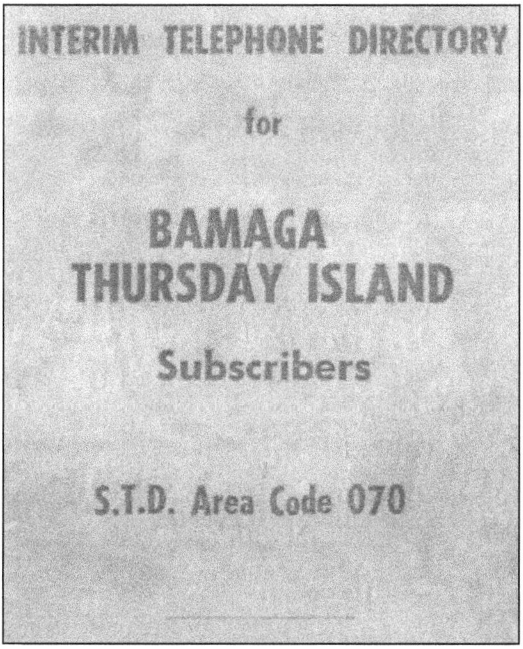

INTERIM TELEPHONE DIRECTORY

for

BAMAGA
THURSDAY ISLAND

Subscribers

S.T.D. Area Code 070

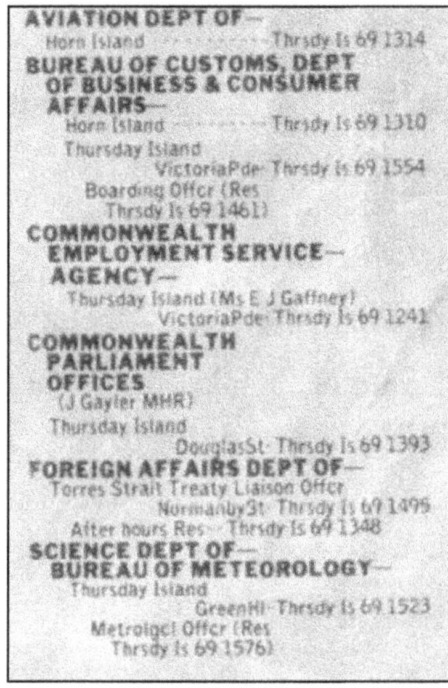

**AVIATION DEPT OF—**
Horn Island ........ Thrsdy Is 69 1314
**BUREAU OF CUSTOMS, DEPT OF BUSINESS & CONSUMER AFFAIRS—**
Horn Island ........ Thrsdy Is 69 1310
Thursday Island
VictoriaPde Thrsdy Is 69 1554
Boarding Offcr (Res Thrsdy Is 69 1461)
**COMMONWEALTH EMPLOYMENT SERVICE— AGENCY—**
Thursday Island (Ms E J Gaffney)
VictoriaPde Thrsdy Is 69 1241
**COMMONWEALTH PARLIAMENT OFFICES**
(J Gayler MHR)
Thursday Island
DouglasSt Thrsdy Is 69 1393
**FOREIGN AFFAIRS DEPT OF—**
Torres Strait Treaty Liaison Offcr
NormanbySt Thrsdy Is 69 1495
After hours Res Thrsdy Is 69 1348
**SCIENCE DEPT OF— BUREAU OF METEOROLOGY—**
Thursday Island
GreenHl Thrsdy Is 69 1523
Metrolgcl Offcr (Res Thrsdy Is 69 1576)

*Cover and page from the Bamaga Interim Telephone Directory, 1983*

and I confided also to Evelyn, Ted and Joe who supported the proposal. That was the last time Joe McGinness and I were actively working together, although he did come up with the Hostel executive team to open the first Jummula Dubbins Hostel. Since then the current hostel is the third.

The Community Chairmen that I had contacted offered their Council Clerks, Yatamo Gela, Langston Nai, Waba Waigana from Saibai and Lilly Ahmat. Our strategy was that I send blank forms to these communities and the council clerks would help the people to register for benefits, and then send their forms to me once a week. I would then send them with my filled forms from Thursday Island to Townsville along with my stats form.

Collectively the registration forms and the statistics collection clarified to the government that there was a great need to establish these offices on Thursday Island to service the Torres Strait for welfare benefits and later CDEP.

I became very unpopular with the Department of Native Affairs, now Family Services, because in their eyes I was encouraging the Islanders to take away the finance which they were handling to their advantage and not to the people's.

As time went on, island after island pulled out of the Department of Native Affairs and registered their people for social benefits through the Department of Social Security and CES.

These services are now called Centrelink and we are forever grateful to the vision of these three people – Joe McGinness, Ted Loban and Evelyn Scott – for pursuing the issue, and the Chairmen – George Mye, Joe Mosby and the late Wagia Waia and Joe Nona – with their council clerks, for being brave and to have taken their people away from the Department of Native Affairs financial system to give them the right to decide their human rights, including women's rights with a single parent pension.

# Health and women's issues

Marjorie Wymarra, an Aboriginal, and Eve Finney, a Maori, formed a Torres Strait Island Women's Association because of homelessness for women and children through domestic violence and lack of accommodation.

Women and children were cared for by these two women and other women helpers in the old picture theatre, as well as from Marjorie Wymarra's home. Marjorie not only was a front runner for women's issues but also for the welfare of Torres Strait people when it was not fashionable for Indigenous people to speak out, especially for a woman, and a black one at that.

Marjorie and Eve came across great difficulties with the Shire Council for having the women and children living in sub-standard circumstances at the old picture theatre and the lack of funds to find the women and children some food. Remember at this time we were only introducing the social benefits through the newly structured Department of Social Security and a Commonwealth Employment Service, so poverty was high.

In June 1988, I came on the scene as a Torres Strait representative for the National Aboriginal Health Strategy Committee which wrote the National Aboriginal Health Strategy report, and invited all women from Torres Strait and the Northern Peninsula Area to attend a women's health meeting on Thursday Island at the Abigail Bann Hostel on the 8th of June 1988.

The women's representatives on the National Aboriginal Health Strategy Committee were all given an area in Australia. Mine obviously was Torres Strait and Northern Peninsula Area (NPA). My duty was to meet with the Aboriginal and Torres Strait women to listen to their views on health issues and services and to set a framework for change to be included in the National Policy on women's health due to be published that year by the Commonwealth Department of Community Services and Health on women's health and to be included in the National Aboriginal Health Strategy Working Party recommendation report.

I invited the women to participate in discussion on education and training for women provided time was available at the meeting. The women's health meeting was attended by 47 women from Northern Peninsula Area to Boigu and across the Torres Strait. Women's health was based on a report by the Aboriginal Women's Task Force 1986 Report by the Office of Status of Women (OSW) and the National Policy on Women's Health 1988.

At the June meeting we were giving our Torres Strait women an opportunity to have input on decisions for their health care to increase their participation and decision making process, especially on prevention and primary health care.

The purpose of a National Policy on women's health was proposed in September 1985 at the second national conference in Adelaide attended by 700 women. The conference identified the importance of women's health in the changing society and that women were the main participants of the health system as both consumers and providers.

Up to the 1980s the women were not well represented in senior professional positions or decision making positions. This affected the way the health care system was run, how resources were allocated and how problems were prioritised and identified, because women have special health problems and health needs which are associated with their reproductive system, and sexual and social roles.

Marjorie Wymarra led the women at our Women's Health meeting to talk about gynaecological problems and antenatal issues or the lack of adequate service for their women's business. Other health needs identified were placement care for aged care and mental health care for families with loved ones that needed special care.

The major current problems were domestic violence and diabetes associated with food and nutrition, and quality of lifestyle, as well as homelessness which created environmental health problems and many more health issues.

The women at this meeting used the last two hours for themselves to talk about our women's business. Everyone felt comfortable to participate. However, Marjorie Wymarra from the Torres Strait Women's Association and Lena Passi, President of the Mother's Union of the Church of England Diocese of Carpentaria, were the front runners as movers and shakers to use this forum to write to various government departments.

The Torres Strait women identified a need for further education and consideration of specific health related issues. These women felt there was a need to advise government Ministers of the major need to improve the conditions affecting their lives which could be contributing to some form of health hazards in antenatal, neonatal and postnatal.

First and foremost the women agreed with and supported Marjorie and Lena that a women's organisation must be set up not just for social welfare but as a spokes vehicle for women's affairs. An

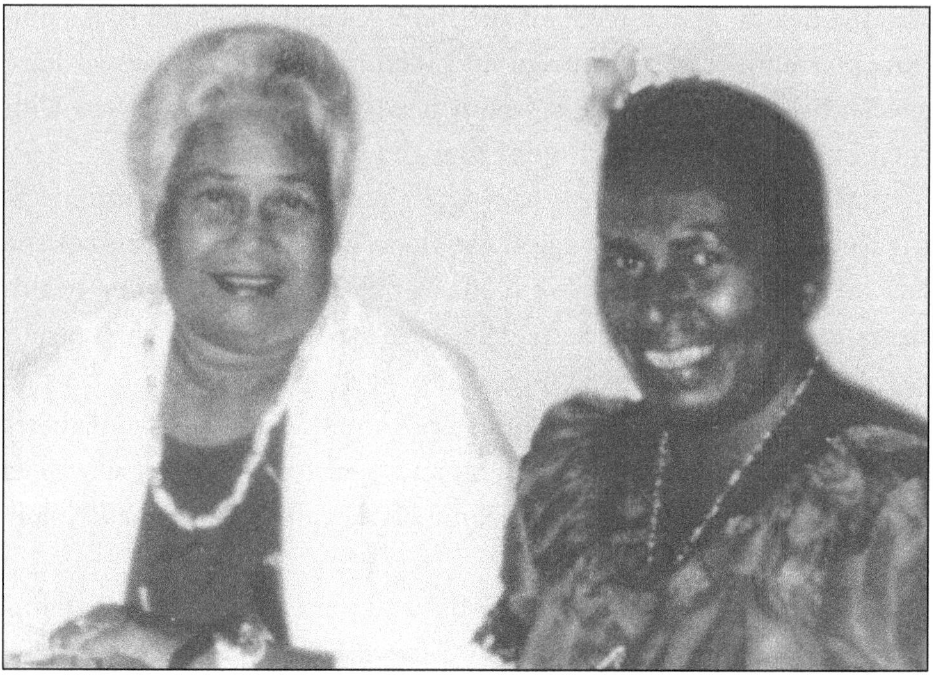

*Ellie Gaffney and Lena Passi, 1988*

interim executive was nominated and elected. I was elected the interim President and Lena Passi my Vice President.

I co-ordinated the meeting because of my role as the Torres Strait representative nominated by the Island Co-ordinating Council Chairman Mr Getano Lui (Jnr) to compile our Torres Strait report on health issues on the National Aboriginal Health Strategy (NAHS).

The NAHS Committee was set up as a working party in December 1987 in Perth at a meeting of Commonwealth, State and Territory ministers responsible for Health and Aboriginal Affairs. This was brought about by Aboriginal and Torres Strait Islander people in regard to their poor health care and delivery.

Health services in the Torres Strait and NPA in those days were fragmented. There were the Bamaga and Thursday Island Hospitals, the Aboriginal Health Team, the State Department Medical Aid Posts, Maternal and Child Welfare and BUAI Alcoholic Program. While the five together were doing a good job, there was very little liaison with each other.

At this meeting the women asked me to make a recommendation for a more effective delivery of care and a more efficient use of people's time. I suggested that an integrated community health service for this area was the only way to go and under a management committee made up of competent local people. This integrated health service was to project relevant training for health workers and enrol nurses aides with qualifications acceptable anywhere in Australia.

The meeting's recommendation for the upgrading of services affecting women's health was to sent to the following people:

The Honourable Gerry Hand, Federal Minister for Aboriginal Affairs
Mr G.C. Jones, Director, Inter Government Relations Branch
The Honourable Lisa Harvey MLA, State Minister for Health
The Honourable J.H. Randall, State Minister for Local Government
Mr Getano Lui (Jnr), Island Co-ordinating Council Chairman and Island Industries Chairman, and
Mr Pat Whelan, Torres Council Shire Clerk.

The meeting also agreed that the next meeting would set up a women's organisation and elect their committee members to seek registration under an act in preparation to achieve the objectives expressed at this meeting, hopefully in their own women's office.

4

# Mura Kosker Sorority

The next time the women met was on the 16th and 17th of August 1988, at the VMI Hall where 36 women attended from the communities representing health workers, education, housewives, community leaders and high school students. The task for this forum was to set aims and objectives for the organisation.

The members elected as committee members were:

| | |
|---|---|
| Ellie Gaffney | President |
| Lena Passi | Vice President |
| Josephine Akee | Secretary/Treasurer |
| Salu Sebasio | Member |
| Lillian Bosun | Member |
| Siai Min | Member |
| Angela Unwin | Member |
| Ethel Banu | Member |
| Waimed Maitie | Member |
| Kailang Dorante | Ex officio Member. |

The aims of the organisation were to work towards uniting women of all ages in the Torres Strait and the NPA and to take steps to meet the social, emotional, housing, educational, economic, health, cultural, spiritual and welfare needs of women and their children/dependants.

The objectives were:

- To participate in the development of all aspects concerning women's issues in Torres Strait and the NPA.
- Greater involvement by women in community concerns in our everyday way of life in Torres Strait and the NPA.
- Identify critical needs and consult and make recommendations to relevant authorities for consideration, approval and implementation.
- To foster self-determination, self-help and self-management and to support groups that are of benefit to women and their families by providing the opportunity to improve work skills in preparation for obtaining employment and promotion to management roles.
- To maintain an interest in the traditional way of life.
- To promote the elimination of discrimination against women.

I raised the matter that we needed to seek legal advice to look at a constitution and register the organisation, which I offered to undertake, and for the women to select a name. The women suggested the word 'Mura' which is a Western Island language meaning 'all of us' and Lena Passi suggested 'Kosker' which was Eastern language meaning 'female'. John Scott suggested the word 'Sorority' meaning 'sisters'.

Hence the organisation became registered as The Mura Kosker Sorority, meaning 'All women are sisters'.

John Scott was a public servant, non-Indigenous, who assisted us in many ways in direction and submission for finance. When we had no money John Scott went as guarantor for our organisation to secure accommodation from See Hop and the promise of paying to enable us to practise for six months.

When the funding came through we had to pay rent arrears for six months as well as wages for the office person I had working with me to bring us up to date. I personally received no money but was kept on when finance came through to establish the organisation and to set up programs and employment services relevant to the aims and objectives.

At this first day of the two-day meeting the Medical Superintendent, Dr Peter Holt, and Registered Nurse, Sandra Kanard, spoke on women's health care and AIDS.

Dr Holt acknowledged that most of the things that were needed regarding health in the Torres Strait had already been covered by the women's recommendation. He went on to say there was the need for more and regular specialist visits by the gynaecologist, paediatrician, ear-nose-and-throat specialist and for increased funding for the hospital. Also the need for Pap Smear tests for our women, with properly equipped facilities, and whom should the attendants be to do the procedure. Bridging the big gap in our district community health centres and social workers was greatly needed.

The women supported Dr Holt's requests and I requested that their recommendations be given to Grace Fischer who, at that time, was the advisor to the State Minister for Health, and Senator Margaret Reynolds of the Office of Status of Women, to brief them. The women were unanimous in making Grace their messenger, because education was taking priority, but we saw that it was now the women's time.

Dr Holt and I projected that the health care most needed was a community health service to be run separately from the hospital service. It should be run by a local board of nine members from the local community. This board was to be involved in the funding for the two services – the hospital and the community health service.

The women's recommendations were given to the doctor to present to the local hospital board to support and forward on to the

Health Department. Included in the recommendation were increased visits by specialists.

A delegation of women attended an ICC meeting to present the women's issues and seek support on a number of issues, including better delivery of goods by cargo vessels to the outer islands by the Island Industries Board, and the role of Department of Native Affairs Medical Aid Posts Health Workers in the community, their employment conditions, the facilities they had to work in and the fact that their hours exceeded their pay rate. The Health Workers were only allowed to work a certain amount of hours and paid accordingly. However, the Health Worker was looking after the whole community and had to stay and finish only when the last patient had been seen. The pay rate was the rate the Department of Native Affairs paid Aboriginals and Torres Strait Islanders living on the community, which was very poor.

Another issue raised from the women's delegation to the ICC was that Health Workers must receive training to give them qualifications, giving them self-esteem and raising their status.

The four women delegation that attended the ICC was myself, Lena Passi, Lillian Bosun and Josephine Akee and there were three of our women on the ICC, Grace Fischer, Chair of St Pauls, Monica Amie and Edna Gebadi, both from NPA.

A letter of support was sent to the Department of Community Services, which was the name change for the Department of Native Affairs, to improve the conditions and wages for the MAP Health Workers.

## Recommendations

A recommendation letter was also sent to the Health Minister, the

Honourable Lisa Harvey, from the women's delegate at the women's health meeting recommending that an integrated community health service was needed in the Torres Strait for a more effective delivery of care and efficient use of people's time. This was emphasised very strongly because of the fragmented services in the district with no real liaison between any of them. The proposed integrated community health care service was to be managed by a management community made up of competent local people. This integrated service was to include every health care provisional unit in the district with a training school on health care similar to the Thursday Island School of Nursing.

Another recommendation was for an immediate appointment of an itinerant Dentist for the Bamaga people and outer island communities, and not to consider them as second priority to the School Dentist which, in the women's opinion, was inadequate.

The women requested a specialist service of visiting sessional specialists for the Thursday Island Hospital as the needs required, especially a Gynaecologist and a domiciliary service similar to the Blue Nursing, with Meals on Wheels as part of the integrated health care centre.

A Family Planning Unit with a female doctor was also requested by the women with competent staff qualified and experienced within this integrated service providing information on contraceptive usage, the types that were available and the quality and their effects.

The women recommended also that a Social Worker be appointed to counsel and work with children and substance abuse victims and any cases with problems related to violence, alcohol and poverty, and for a new Maternal and Child Welfare clinic to be set up on Thursday Island with enough staff to do field work.

Whilst making recommendations is one thing, we needed Health Workers to have adequate training in a mainstream system for better understanding of the human body and its physiology as well for the Health Worker to receive training and qualification to register under a State board enabling them to be accepted when moving around in employment like any other Australians.

The meeting argued that the educational program to be implemented must be continual to the providers of health care on AIDS, Diabetes, Heart Disease and others as required in a teaching manner relevant to the race of people who are the recipients.

The women requested the Health Workers be trained to do Pap Smears and breast examinations and funding be allocated for their training and for more trained nurses to be placed on the outer islands and for a community-based TAFE course training in Health Care to be on Thursday Island.

The women requested priority staff accommodation for southern and local health workers on Thursday Island and outer islands and that the MAP services be 24 hours, and to install a 24-hour telephone service with an alarm system as well the need for doctors to visit the communities fortnightly instead of monthly.

The women requested that the Minister consider having competent women on the Hospital board as a priority.

I now bring the readers up to date on whether any of these recommendations were followed up and established.

The request on women's business firstly was Dr Holt's dilemma because of the increased death rate of our women from cancer of the reproductive organs. Together with one of our Indigenous Health Workers, Yoko Nakata, he undertook to set up a clinic under a specialised service clinic to do Pap Smears.

Yoko went away to get training and an external course on women's health and Dr Holt went to Sheffield, UK, to train to do Colposcopy.

Yoko received her diploma in sexual health and became the program co-ordinator for the Men's and Women's Health Program for the Torres Strait and NPA district.

Between them, Dr Holt and Yoko perfected the women's health program with effective clinics and colposcopy done regularly as well as Pap Smears and men's and women's education on their health care. These two wonderful caring people have made a tremendous impact on the women and their families' lives. Fewer women are dying now because the problem is detected earlier, allowing something to be done.

Dr Holt received the Queen's Honours Award for his pioneering work in Torres Strait Islands women's health and Yoko is studying to become a registered nurse.

Colposcopy is now done by a female doctor and there are two other female doctors who can relieve, whilst Yoko, in the midst of running her very busy program, has trained our Indigenous staff to do the clinics and the Colposcopy with the doctors.

What a wonderful thing these two people did answering the Torres Strait women's prayer and the request by Lena Passi and Marjorie Wymarra at the Women's Health Meeting in June 1988.

Dr Peter Holt first came to the Torres Strait in June 1973 with his family, his wife, Pat, and three young children 30 years ago. Dr Holt has worked tirelessly for the people in caring and introducing many programs for our benefits. That is another story someone should write about this wonderful doctor. He is truly a legend and he is still working physically and promoting programs for better health for our

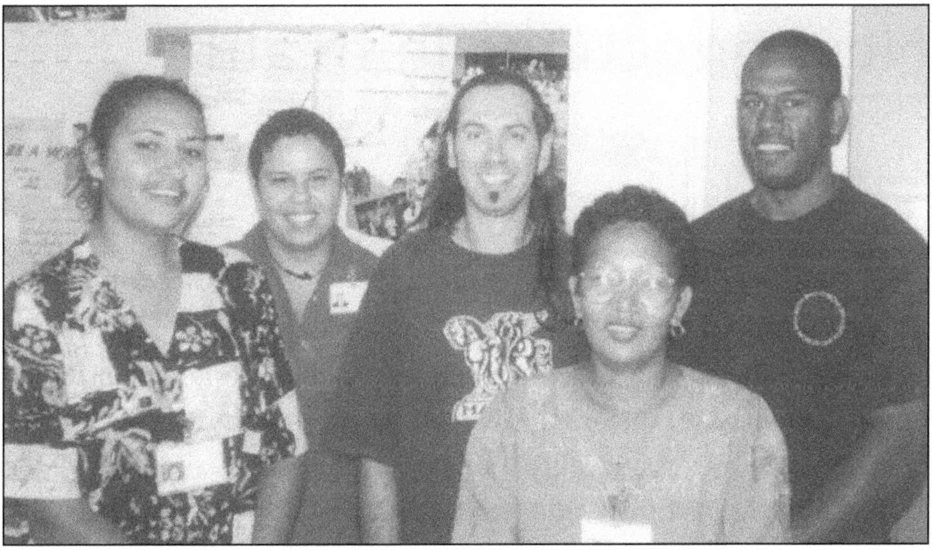

*Yoko Nakata (front) with the Men's and Women's Health Team*

people. It will be a very sad day when he leaves us to retire. However, he is overdue to spend some time with his family, especially his wife who has allowed him the time to look after us. Holty, we will miss you when you go away. God's blessing to Pat and you.

5

# New directions in health

One of the women's requests to Lisa Harvey, the State Minister for Health, was to consider having a competent local woman on the hospital board as a priority. Well, things were going in a different direction for Queensland public sector health services and in 1990 the Queensland Department of Health produced a green paper to give information to the community about a proposal for change. The government was considering making hospital boards redundant, amongst other things, and the green paper was really a discussion paper directed by the government purely for discussion by the people. The State Health Minister was then Ken McElligott MLA.

A group of us on Thursday Island got together to peruse the green paper. We met a few times to set out our comments and submission relating to our health needs and other matters relating to the green paper, and this was sent on to the Department of Health for consideration.

One of the requests was to replace the Hospital Board with a District Health Council. This request was approved and Grace Fischer was made the Chairperson of the Health Council in the Torres Strait sector. She held that position for twelve years.

I believe the first thing Grace did was to lobby with the Island Co-ordinating Councils and Chairman Mr Getano Lui Jnr to second Mr Phillip Mills from the Office of Torres Strait Islander Affairs

Secretariat in Canberra. The request was supported and approved by the Federal Minister for Aboriginal Affairs.

The secondment employed Phillip Mills as District Manager for two years to develop health services throughout the Torres Strait and NPA. Together with Grace Fischer they made a good team during the development in rebuilding the third Thursday Island Hospital after the first post war hospital and also a Primary Health Care Centre to separate the health services into acute care at the hospital and non acute in prevention and education at the Primary Health Care Centre.

Phillip was seconded for two years and after over a decade he is still here working for the district. Grace has moved back to her community, St Paul's on Moa Island, to perhaps get back her life after working voluntarily for other people for twelve years. However she is still working tirelessly amongst her people and studying at the same time.

During the development Phillip and Grace contracted a Fijian Doctor, Elekana Faafoi, as the Director of Primary Health Care, and I was employed shortly after to do some work in Diabetes, and later to set up and work in the new Primary Health Care Centre as the Health Centre Manager.

Dr Elekana, with the District Manager, developed the Torres Strait Model for Primary Health Care. In this model were the thirteen essential health care services identified by the Torres Strait Health Strategy. This Strategy was co-ordinated by the District Manager in a workshop to provide and inform the community of priorities impacting on the health status of the Torres Strait and Northern Peninsula Area people. This workshop was held in 1993 giving recognition to the National Aboriginal Health Strategy report (NAHS) that the people maintain a cultural heritage which demanded that, when developing health programs for us, consideration must be given to maintain at all times culturally appropriate service programs.

In the Torres Strait Health Strategy (see Appendix), the people sought community empowerment by provision of more community based health care activities and encouragement of community involvement and participation in the health care action.

Dr Elekana structured a guide on the development of Primary Health Care services in the Torres District based on reports from:

- 1989 The National Aboriginal Health Strategy
- 1992 Queensland Primary Health Care Policy
- 1993 Torres Strait Health Strategy
- 1994 Queensland Aboriginal and Torres Strait Islander Health Policy
- 1996 The Implementation Plan of the Torres Strait Health Strategy
- 1997 The Development of the Torres Strait Model for Primary Health Care by the PHC Management Team and the development of the Torres Strait PHC Planning Matrix, and operational procedures and case management and development of program specific work plans
- 1998 The development of position description and duty statements for Indigenous Primary Health Centre management and operational staff.

The thirteen essential health care services identified by the Torres Strait Health Strategy were renamed as Program Areas and were delivered using the Torres Strait model for Primary Health Care.

The areas are Primary Health Care, Post Acute and Rehabilitation, Child Care Women's Health, Sexual Health, Communicable

Disease Control, Alcohol and Drug Control, Mental Health, Social/ Family Health, Oral/Dental Health, Hearing Health and Environmental Health.

A Program Co-ordinator position was established to run the programs which were divided into five services to implement and for the selection of the right person for the job, and also avoidance of waste through duplication, and maintenance of a harmonious working relationship between clients and health workers.

The integrated services were Primary Health Care, Screening and Prevention, Health Education, Health Promotion and Community Development.

## Primary care

The Integrated Service was to provide 100 per cent GP Practice and 24 hours Accident and Emergency Service and acute care, and to employ more doctors.

## Screening and prevention

To provide health screening and referral service to program areas co-ordinated 75 per cent by health workers and to include the people concerned by 25 per cent.

## Health education

Responsibilities are shared by Health Workers and Clients, Health Workers to educate and clients to accept responsibilities for their health care.

## Health promotion

Promote access to Primary Clinical Care by the community and the importance of early presentation for treatment. Develop resources to support services. The health workers responsibility is 25 per cent and 75 per cent is the responsibility of the clients.

## Community development and empowerment

The responsibility was to empower the community 100 per cent to establish their own community based health care centres, with 100 per cent involvement and participation in health care action.

The Women's Health and other health needs recommended by the Women's meeting were almost completed by the development and as a result of the efforts of people like the District Manager, Grace Fischer, Dr Holt and Dr Elekana.

Dr Elekana left the development after three years in the Torres Strait. I believe he has gone back to study, but still has an interest in the outer island health programs.

The heavenly Father was good to the Torres Strait by bringing the right people up at the right time and place.

6

# Domestic violence

Mura Kosker Sorority was now incorporated under the Queensland Associations Act. Its office was in Douglas Street, rented off Mrs Phyllis Ahloy of See Hop & Co.

Together with the management committee, I set up six programs to be managed by our organisation: the Mura Kosker Sorority Domestic Violence Program, the Home and Community and Care Program, the OPAP Program for the aged, the Emergency Relief Fund for people in crises, RAATSICC program for childcare and the Special Projects Program to raise funds for women to travel and attend women's meetings State-wide, Nationally and Internationally.

Domestic violence is experienced by people of every age group and from all cultures, religion, and socio-economic, educational and occupational backgrounds.

The Mura Kosker Sorority Domestic Violence Program was established because of the violence in the families. Victims were powerless and were abused physically, verbally and sexually, resulting in psychological problems with financial hardship and/or homelessness.

The role of Mura Kosker Sorority firstly is to secure a safe place for the women, and children if there are children involved. Sometimes the women may have to go to the hospital for treatment, or admission if the injury is serious; then the woman is taken to the Police Station to take out a protection order to go to court.

Many of the women are very nervous because they have never

been to court before. The perpetrator usually has a solicitor and the police act on behalf of the women victims. The women then have to be taken to the Department of Social Security. At that time there was a draft National Policy Statement on Domestic Violence and the Department of Social Security was to support the victims of domestic violence. In the past they have had cases where people have had to be evacuated down south. It can be very difficult to organise to get people out of the outer islands.

It was a mammoth task trying to co-ordinate all the organisations or agents working together to assist the Domestic Violence victims.

The safe places were in a Mura Kosker Sorority member's home, hospital or evacuation to south. This actually strengthened the women's case to establish a women's shelter on Thursday Island. It was important to get an approach and work out the situation and we treated each situation on its own merit.

Some of the Domestic Violence cases were men, so I employed an Indigenous male Domestic Violence Officer. Kenny Bedford was the first male Indigenous Domestic Violence Officer and the second male Domestic Violence Officer in Queensland; the first was a non-Indigenous male.

The Department of Social Security had a standard procedure for dealing with domestic violence matters and they were given priority, for example, addresses and information kept confidential with limited access to files thus lessening the leaking of information. To lessen financial hardship, special benefits could be made available, with maintenance to be taken out against the perpetrator. Benefits usually going to the husband were now split and many more assistances were available.

A select committee from Mura Kosker Sorority members formed a planning committee for the women's shelter and has been in opera-

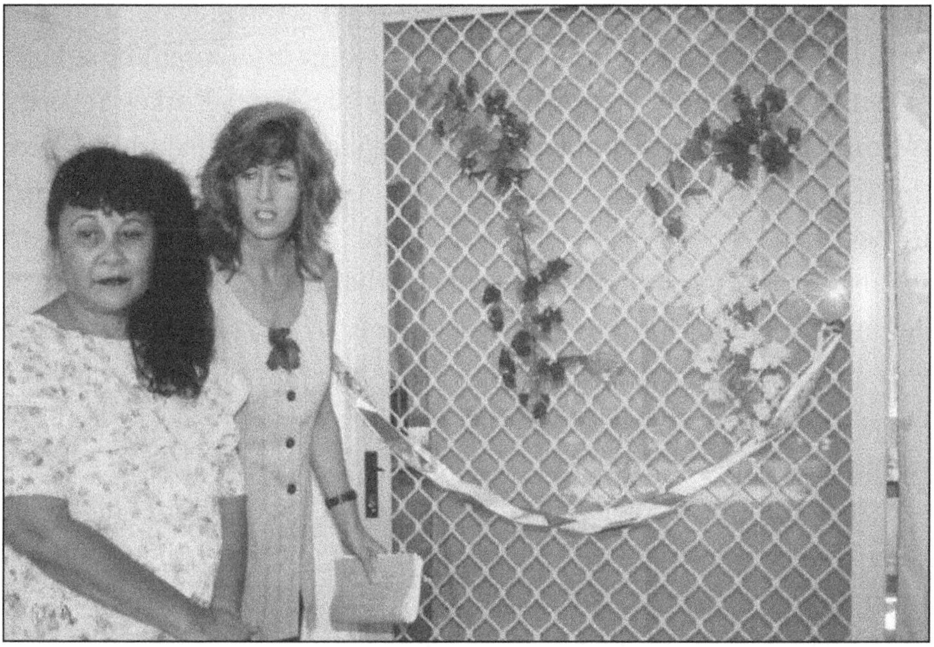

*Mura Solwata Kosker President Jenny Vellis and Vice-President Val Schier officially open the Lena Passi Women's Shelter*

tion since 1990 and we had written three submissions to the Department of Family Service for funding to build the shelter and eventually we were successful in getting an allocation of $250,000 in June 1992. Our planning committee, made up of Val Schier, Ellie Gaffney, Lena Passi (until she died on the 14th of September 1992), Jenny Vellis, Louise Ghee and Elaine Bin Juda held many sessions to decide what should go into the shelter.

The Department of Family Services offered their services to assist in the design of the building and organising tenders and supervising construction of the shelter as they had done at Bamaga.

There were many frustrations as the first design originally proved to be too expensive and we had to start from scratch again. Then we were advised that nothing could go ahead as the land might be subject to native land claim. I then took it on as the Mura Kosker Sorority Co-ordinator to make contact with the Department of Family Services for Aboriginal & Islander Affairs Minister Anne Warner and explained to her that I would like an appointment to see her. She agreed to see me for half an hour between her parliamentary sittings the next day in Brisbane. This was not much time, so I arranged a meeting with representatives of the traditional Kaurareg owners to explain our needs and why we needed to build a shelter for the protection of the women and children.

The traditional owners agreed to allow us to build the shelter on their land; however should the status of usage change then the land must be given back. They gave me a letter on their letterhead to show to the Minister Anne Warner and I booked myself on the morning flight out of Horn Island to Brisbane to get me there on time to meet with the Minister.

Whilst I was waiting on Horn Island to fly out, one of the southern Department of Family Services Officers arrived on the incoming plane. We greeted and she enquired as to where I was going and when I told her she actually burst out laughing and said, 'What do you think she can do?' I just looked at her.

I arrived in Brisbane on time, checked into the Bellevue Hotel and caught a taxi to the Parliament House. Minister Warner was there with her Secretary, an officer from the Land Commission and her Legal Advisor. I showed her the Kaurareg traditional owners' letter and in half an hour the bell rang for her to return to sitting, but not before she approved and then advised her team to proceed with the letter of approval to go ahead with the building.

On my return to Thursday Island, I advised the planning committee of our success so the Department of Family Services for Aboriginal & Islander Affairs would award the tender the same week and construction may be completed that year, depending on the wet. The shelter was built on the land next to the Police Station so it should be safe.

When the shelter was built it was a double storey building. The staffing was two full time Domestic Violence Officers, a male and a female, a part time caretaker and Admin was from the Mura Kosker Sorority office to save administration costs, and volunteers were put on a rotating relieving roster to give a 24-hour service. This shelter was named after Lena Passi for her contribution towards the women's movement and later another building was built next to the

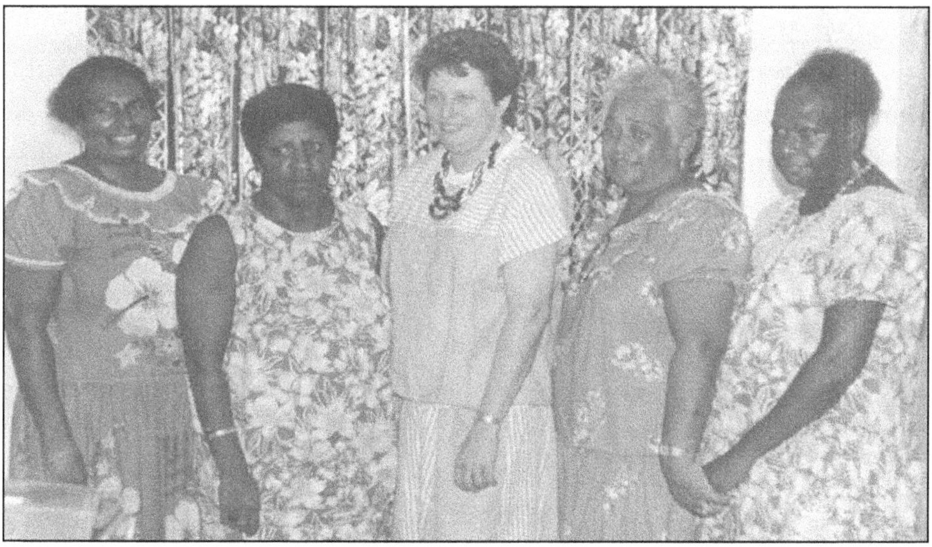

*Northern Peninsular Area Women, Margie Daniels and Monica Unwin with Lena Passi and Ellie Gaffney at the Shelter's Opening, with Jan Williams, Under-Secretary, TATSIC, Department of Family Services*

shelter and was named after the other woman mover and shaker, Marjorie Gwendoline Wymarra.

The Lena Passi shelter was opened and blessed by Lena's husband, David Passi. I didn't invite the Department of Family Services Officer who scoffed at me on Horn Island to the opening even though she was the officer who funded Mura Kosker Sorority through the SAAP program.

This officer, at a later date after my time, was instrumental in splitting the shelter from its founder, the Mura Kosker Sorority. The women suspected that it was a move to enable a person of her choice and an employee of the Lena Passi Shelter (and encouraged by that person) to stay employed while standing for office at Mura Kosker Sorority and/or vice versa – because the funding body sponsor's policy was that an employee of an organisation could only be one or the other and not both.

This was a very bad and irresponsible decision; it stopped the women's movement in its tracks and fragmented the women's unity. If we were going to decrease domestic violence then it was vital that everyone worked together for all women from all walks of life in the Torres Strait and not for cliques of people and nepotism by state government officers.

The State Government of that time found it very difficult to accept that women, especially Aboriginal and Torres Strait Islander women, could run their own affairs. During the early times of Mura Kosker Sorority formation, the Queensland Health Department sent a team of women doctors and registered nurses from Brisbane to advise the health workers here on 'women's health' and management.

They held their meeting at the CWA Hall in Douglas Street at the top end and, at the time, the Mura Kosker Sorority women were hold-

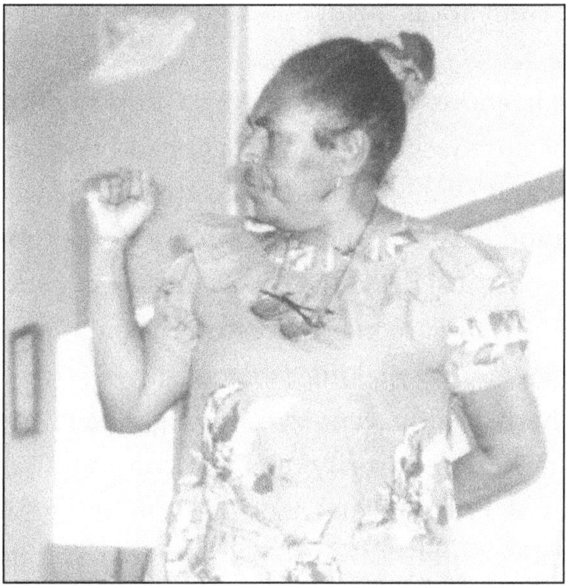

*The late Lena Passi tells the Queensland Health Department meeting, CWA Hall, Thursday Island: 'Nobody make decision for my health, except me.'*

ing their annual general meeting at Mura Mudh Hostel on Douglas Street at the bottom end. When the news got to us – that this delegation of women in Health from Brisbane was on Thursday Island and holding a meeting on our health – anger broke out amongst the women at the thought that the southern health team would come to our island and ignore Mura Kosker Sorority who made the recommendations. So our women stopped our meeting and hopped into three vans and drove up to the other meeting. We walked in and took over, saying that the meeting, as far as the Torres Strait women were concerned, was invalid. Lena Passi said, 'Nobody make decision for my health, except me.'

The poor women from the south appeared upset because they

had breeched our local protocol for consultation and perhaps negotiation.

A non-Indigenous member of Mura Kosker Sorority who is a registered nurse approached me and suggested I try and compromise. So I stepped in and explained to the meeting of the women that culturally they should have consulted with Mura Kosker Sorority because in the NAHS report it states our people must be consulted before any decisions on our health are made, because consultation is the essential component of any policy making or decisions.

The southern health team was leaving TI the next day, so the women of Mura Kosker Sorority offered a compromise joint meeting under the trees at Friday Island that day and all agreed. The Torres Strait Co-operative barge 'Kalyara' was chartered and the women had their meeting at Friday Island and a late barbecue lunch before returning to TI that afternoon. At the meeting the TSI & NPA women asked for an itinerant midwife for the outer islands and to raise the specific women's health services to meet the TSI & NPA women's needs that had never been considered before. These requests were approved.

Lena Passi didn't make it to the next annual general meeting. As previously mentioned, she passed away on the 14th of September 1992, just before she was due to return to TI.

I usually put in long hours at the office each day, Monday to Friday, 8 a.m. to 6.30 p.m., and the afternoon before her death, at 6 p.m., I received a phone call at the office from her. Lena advised me that she was coming into TI the next day on the eleven o'clock ferry and she would be attending the annual general meeting before flying out to a Church of England Mothers' Union meeting down south.

I offered that we would meet the eleven o'clock ferry and treat her to lunch at the Mura Kosker Sorority office before checking her into the accommodation. The next day when Lena was due, I was awakened at 7 a.m. by my husband who advised me that a message had come through for me that Lena Passi had passed away and that the family would be bringing her body into TI on the eleven o'clock ferry.

I was stunned because she did come on the eleven o'clock ferry like she told me, but not alive. I missed her then and still reflect with sadness because Lena and I go back some time. We used to nurse together at the TI and Waiben Hospitals.

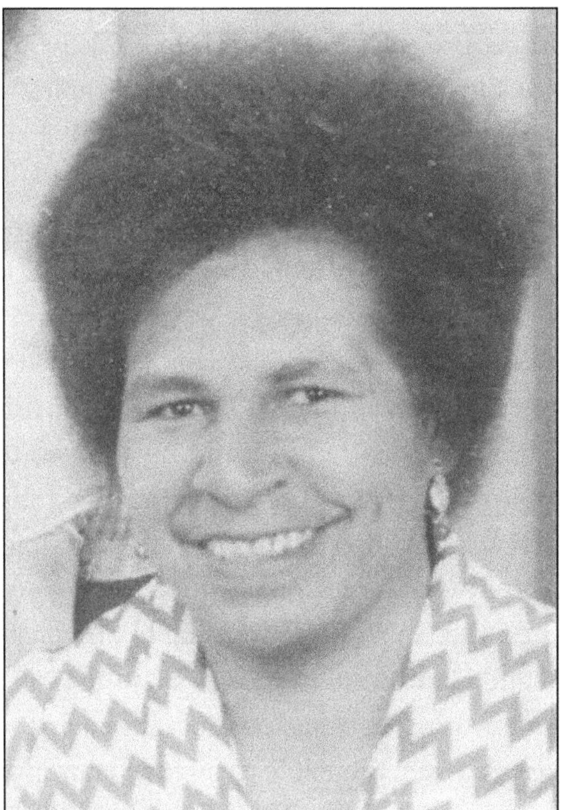

*The late Lena Passi*

7

# Health services in the Torres Strait

The Home and Community Care (HACC) service was a service the Mura Kosker Sorority provided to the frail aged and disabled people. This program was brought to our attention by the State Health, Aboriginal Health Program and the Mura Kosker Sorority Secretary. Josephine Akee did the submission and we applied to manage the service for our old people and we were successful.

The Qld State Health funded Mura Kosker Sorority, but very poorly. However we provided the basic support services in home helpers, transport for clients to health appointments, shopping and banking. We did home visits once a week to Horn, Hammond and Thursday Islands. At first, Louise Ghee and I included the visits as part of our duty to cut down on the costs until we got funding for a part time co-ordinator and then Louise's and my job was to raise the extra funding to employ that HACC Co-ordinator on a full time basis.

Our first HACC Co-ordinator was Kura Stephen and then Keith Fell followed. Both were exceptionally good, caring and efficient.

Louise and I then applied for funding to purchase a dinghy to use to get to Horn and Hammond Islands so that the HACC Co-ordinator could visit as many old people as possible instead of being tied to the ferry timetables. We were then able to include Hammond Island in the visits. The team effort here was unbelievable work-wise and raising funds to promote and streamline the services for our aged people.

We then introduced Meals on Wheels for one meal a day cooked by the TI Hospital and delivered to our oldies at home. Day respite was provided wherever they wished, usually at the Star of the Sea Home for the Aged or Thursday Island Hospital.

The hospital provided a different respite for clients because their homes weren't built to cater for aged and/or disabled and the hospital staff bathed and shampooed the client's hair and provided meals as well as having the doctor on duty to do an assessment, which to our thinking was a day well spent. The Ambulance provided the pick up and drop off usually because of the difficulty of the HACC Co-ordinator to manage these high maintenance cases by himself.

Working together with the Torres Strait Housing Co-operative, the home's modification structural changes were made.

The HACC Co-ordinator and Mura Kosker Sorority office staff worked together to provide social recreations jointly with OPAP, the Old People's Action Program for active aged folks. I brought this service into Mura Kosker Sorority to work jointly with HACC to compliment each other and to give our aged people more support with a variety of socials like BBQs, card evenings, competition in playing Jaro, movies of Thursday Island or Torres Strait, dancing competition, Keno and other social recreation as well as other services already mentioned that HACC was involved in.

HACC was available Monday to Friday, 9 a.m. to 4 p.m. When the HACC Co-ordinator was visiting Horn and Hammond Islands, other office staff filled in. It was a community service that Mura Kosker Sorority provided during my time to give our senior citizens a voice instead of being a silent population of our area.

When we established our HACC services, I encouraged NPA to establish HACC for NPA through the Director of Nursing of the

Bamaga Hospital who negotiated with the Community Council and jointly they established theirs, then the Island Co-ordinating established theirs to service the other islands.

Shortly after, Mura Kosker Sorority was approached to take on the Emergency Relief funds because the current agent was running into difficulty with the financial management. Mura Kosker Sorority took it on, which proved a tremendous help to low income earners and domestic violence victims.

Whilst we were looking after the aged, we observed that there was a great need for suitable accommodation for our elderly because the homes they were living in were overcrowded and not suitable for aged and/or disabled, with no hand rails, ramp, bathroom with shower recess for the aged. Later the Catholic Church took over the nurses' quarters at Waibene where the Waibene Chest Hospital used to be. They turned it into a place for some of the elderly that was low maintenance and could only take in up to ten to twelve clients because of limited beds and staff.

The Catholic Church aged care home was called the 'Star of the Sea', which I'm told is the meaning of *Stella Maris* in Latin, a spiritual name, because the home was on the side of the sea. The Church's only income was from donations and a small grant from the DNA. The Handmaidens of the Lord worked tirelessly and voluntarily. Catholic women put in time voluntarily and a very few staff were on a low payroll.

These were committed people even though employed on low payroll or voluntary. They committed themselves to the cause. Rev. Fr Mullins and Sister Elva were two of these people who, in my opinion, were saints for the long hours they put into the aged home and running this establishment on the smell of an oily rag.

8

# A new aged-care hostel

One day Fr Mullins called into Mura Kosker Sorority office to see me and I was saddened to see him looking depressed and ready to give up the battle because of lack of funds to continue, in spite of his effort to seek funding from all over the place.

I suggested to Father to perhaps close the place down if his peers allowed it and to place our elderlies in the hospital for care until something could be done. This eventuated and the Medical Superintendent, Dr Peter Holt, called in to see me, a little reluctant about allowing acute beds to be filled by aged care and about how long these elderlies would be in hospital. (It was actually something like three years that they were at the TI Hospital.)

When the elderlies were placed in the hospital, a group of people was formed as the working party to secure funding to build an aged home and for commissioning with staff and equipment. We had to secure the land because of once again the native title issue. We met with the same traditional owners, the Kaurareg representatives, and approval was given again on their letterhead for usage of that land for an aged home for our people. However, should the status of usage change, the land would be handed back to them.

In a planning process meeting to establish this aged persons home, the committee agreed to seek expert advice from George James, an Architect, because of his experience in establishing aged homes in far north Queensland. We seconded George James firstly as a friend and advisor, then later as the Architect of the Home.

The formation and establishment planning eventuated from the Mura Kosker Sorority office where the seed was first planted. By this time, I was no longer the President of Mura Kosker Sorority because of the funding body's policy that one is either a management committee member or employee, not both.

So I became the Co-ordinator for Mura Kosker Sorority, Louise Ghee the Administrator and Jenny Vellis the President when I stepped down. The three of us were part of the foundation members of the aged home. The others were Dr Peter Holt, Fr Mullins, Kathy Cook (Registered Nurse), Jim Akee, Romina Fujii and Lully Filewood. We formed the working committee.

The actual beginning of the thought originated in 1989. George James did the negotiation with government bodies for funding and wrote up the submission seeking funds and eventually $4.6 million was promised by the Commonwealth. Then George James drafted a plan which included a nursing wing and because of this and the Commonwealth lack of trust and vision that locals were capable of overseeing and managing an aged home with a nursing wing, the money promised was put on hold. This poor vision of the Commonwealth public servant officers created hardship for the committee which was made up of qualified health care people with experience.

George James and Mura Kosker Sorority secured funding and sent a delegation of George and some of the committee members to Alice Springs to check out the 'Hetti Perkins' home for the Aged that had a nursing wing.

On their return Jim Akee and George James reported that perhaps we should seek Aboriginal Hostels Limited assistance, just like

Hetti Perkins Home did. This we did and AHL gave a promise of $200,000, then on the eleventh hour they pulled out. This money was to assist us in the initial stage, as a kick start. But when we started we had a deficit of $200,000.

However, after George James negotiated again with the Commonwealth on our behalf, the funding came through. All this process eventuated out of the Mura Kosker Sorority office approved by the President of the Mura Kosker Sorority Jenny Vellis. We used their infrastructure to set up the aged home.

In 1991 as the President of the aged home, I wrote to Mark Stower, Solicitor, to advise him that at the committee meeting in October 1991, the committee passed a special resolution under Section 28 of the Associations Incorporation Act that we apply to the Under Secretary for approval to alter the rules of the Association regarding membership of the management committee as follows:

> *Clause 11(1)* The Management Committee of the Association shall consist of a President, Vice President, Secretary and Treasurer, all of whom shall be members of the Association and such members of the association, so as the total twelve (12) members on the management committee.
>
> *Clause 11(2)* At the first Annual General Meeting of the Association, six (6) members of the management committee for the time being shall retire from office and at the AGM in each subsequent year, the Directors shall retire in rotation of six (6) and six (6) but all returning members shall be eligible upon nomination for re-election.
>
> *Clause 11(3)* same as in present rules.
>
> *Clause 12* same as in present rules.

Thus the Aged Home was incorporated and renamed the Star of the Sea, and the Management Committee elected as follows:

| | |
|---|---|
| Ellie Gaffney | President |
| Lully Filewood | Vice President |
| Dr Peter Holt | Secretary |
| Fr Tom Mullins | Treasurer. |

Members who served from time to time were Romina Fujii, Louise Ghee, Jenny Vellis, Jim Akee, Kathy Cook, John Majid, Dalton Bon, Josephine Akee, Carol Thompson, Agnes Fox, Tassie McDonald, Helen Barrett, Caroline Cloudy, Leanne Chandler, Tracey and Kevin Fujii, Tony Gaffney, George Dewis, Edward Wymarra, Janet Benson and Vicky Tamwoy.

It was six years from the time of incorporation until the home was ready to open on the 26th of October 1995. This was because of hiccups from, firstly. the government and their officers with their stop-start with the promised money. Prices were increasing but the grant remained the same and we had extra expenses like the Ergon cost for installation of power supply which originally was $29,000 but had rocketed to $160,000, which was an extra $131,000 we had to find. The committee went back to the drawing board with the architect and we decided to forego the recreation gazebo that was planned to be built between the hostel and the nursing wing for an entertaining area for the clients instead of sitting under the lean-to or just watching TV in the dining room as they did at the time.

Another sacrifice was when the sullage connection increased and still the grant remained the same. So we had to take away the air-conditioning from the hostel and the Architect had to change his drawings and plumbing plans . George went through all these changes

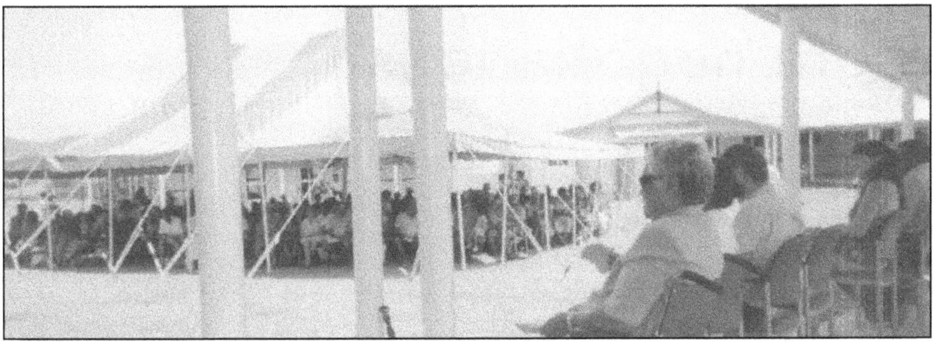

*Star of the Sea Home for the Aged opening day*

but never charged us extra. He stuck to the budget and built this aged home for the $4.6 million.

The Home is a complex consisting of a 15-bed nursing wing, and a 25-bed hostel for a different category of clients as well as four independent living units for a far more independent aged client and perhaps a carer. We refurbished the nuns' accommodation to accommodate three registered nurses. The hostel has three suites to accommodate couples and has three two-bedroom units with kitchen facilities and ensuites.

The nursing wing comprises of one single bedroom and three twin-share rooms and two four-bed wards, each with adjoining toilets and shower facilities.

But once again the building was put on hold by the Shire Council, this time because they felt the size of the home would have a higher consumption of water and at that time water was very scarce, so no new buildings were allowed to be built if there were no pre-existing water services on the land. In the aged home issue, the problem was that we would have a higher consumption of water.

9

# More negotiations

Mura Kosker Sorority sent Flo Kennedy and me to Canberra to a National Women's meeting because we were the two Torres Strait women who went to Africa for the 1985 'End of the Decade' Conference for Women. But we had another mission on our agenda.

We knew the Federal Minister for Local Government, Ms Wendy Fatin, would be at the conference because she was also the Minister advising the Prime Minister on the Office of Status of Women.

Flo and I saw Minister Fatin the first day at the conference and during the lunch break, we sat with her and discussed all the grievances we took down with us, like the unsealed road in front of the Bamaga Hospital and between St Paul's and Kubin communities, the hold up of the aged home and that the aged clients were occupying acute beds at the TI Hospital, as well the illegal immigrants from PNG and other things. Minister Fatin assured Flo and I that she would come up to TSI as soon as possible after she took her mum to Port Douglas for some quality time together. That she did and we accommodated her at the 'Four Winds' overnight and on the afternoon of her arrival, we took her to the Aged Home site then onto the TI Hospital to see the elderlies. Minister Fatin became emotional when she saw them being cared for as acute cases instead of like the aged should be cared for.

A couple of the Mura Kosker Sorority women, Grace Fischer among them, spent the night at the 'Four Winds' to keep the Minister and her Secretary company. The next morning we flew out to Bamaga.

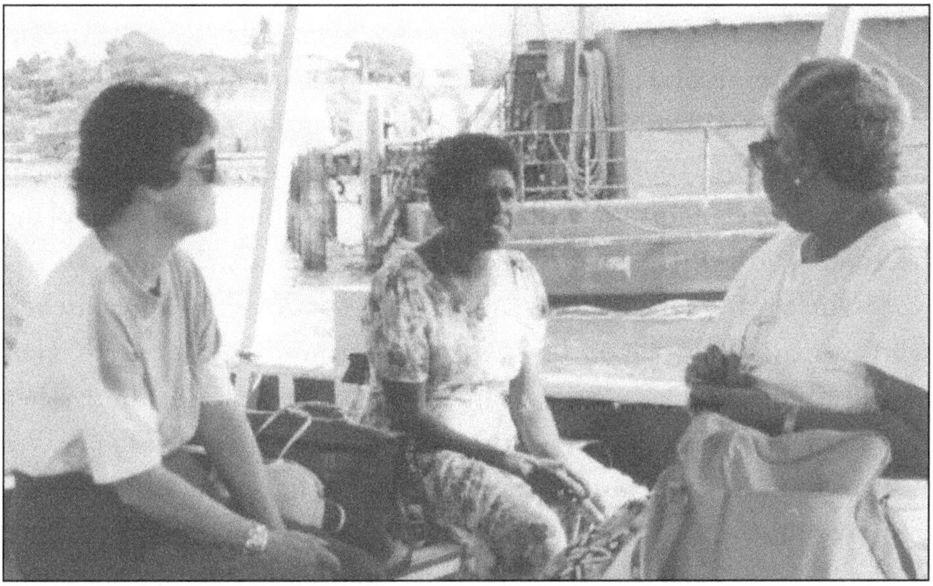

*Federal Minister for Local Government and Minister advising the Prime Minister on the Office of Status of Women, Wendy Fatin with Grace Fisher and Ellie Gaffney en route to Bamaga and Moa*

She flew in her plane and Mura Kosker Sorority chartered a plane for us. We were met by the NPA women from their women's organisation who took us in a bus to Injinoo and Umagico and past the Bamaga Hospital. The NPA women gave us lunch and then we flew to Moa Island and drove on to St Paul's by road.

That evening Grace Fischer arranged a meeting after a feast of a dinner and the Minister listened to the women and her Secretary documented the women's business. Mostly their concern was for a sealed road or a helicopter service for medivac, or both, and to assist in raising the status of women in the Torres Strait, especially in overcoming domestic violence.

The next morning, the Minister was to continue onto Boigu and

Saibai to check out the illegal immigrants issue because she came up under five ministerial portfolios, her two and the Aboriginal Affairs, Health and Immigration portfolios. She didn't make it to Boigu because the first war on Iraq happened and all Ministers were recalled to Parliament in Canberra so we had to get her to Kubin to catch her plane because, as you would have guessed, there was no airstrip at St Paul's.

Our convoy left St Paul's after saying goodbye to Grace Fischer, who was the Chairperson of St Paul's community at that time. Half way to Kubin, Minister Fatin's vehicle broke down, so we bundled her into ours and we went on foot until the vehicle came back for us. We just got to the airport in time to wave to her as her plane taxied on the runway outward. She later wrote to Mura Kosker Sorority thanking us for looking after her and the experience, and that when she speaks in Parliament about the issues in Torres Strait we raised, it would be with experience.

When she was at the 'Four Winds', we had filled empty cordial bottles with rainwater from the tank and she enquired as to what was in the bottles. 'It's drinking water for you' was our reply. She said when she returned to Canberra and allocated funds to the Queensland Minister for Local Government she would make mention of our Shire's water problem and would request that the aged home be allowed to be built, whatever happened. Whether or not Minister Fatin was influential, our aged home got the go ahead because water was going to be pumped to TI from Horn Island, the road between Kubin and St Paul's was sealed and St Paul's has a helicopter pad for helicopter service and the road in front of the Bamaga Hospital is now sealed.

The aged home took eighteen months to build.

Before we could build we had to do a lot of levelling and filling of the site and soil testing and the sea level was measured. That's why we

## Star of the Sea Keys Handed Back to Committee

Last Wednesday the keys for the Star of the Sea Home for the Aged were handed back to the Committee in a short ceremony outside of the new building.

Peter Mathews from P. & E. Mathews Construction Pty Ltd and Mr George James from James Architects handed the keys back to Mrs Ellie Gaffney, the Chairperson for the Committee of the Home for the Aged.

The short ceremony was attended by the members of the committee and Staff Consultant Mr Warren Hann.

The Home for the Aged is expected to officially open at the end of October, with advertising for staff already underway.

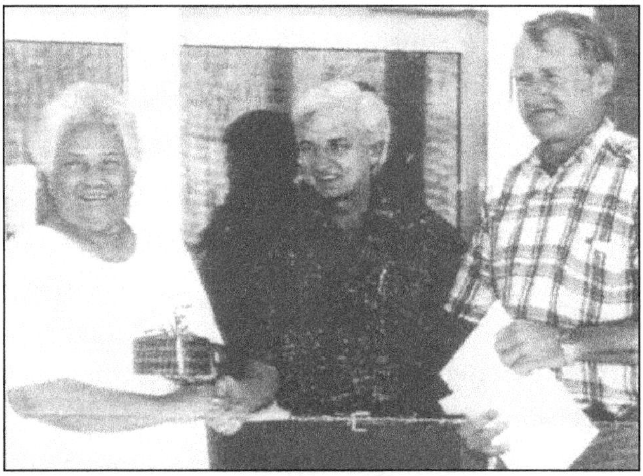

*'Star of the Sea Keys Handed Back to Committee':*
*Ellie Gaffney with George James (centre) and Peter Mathews*

*Source*: *Torres News*, 18–24 August 1995

raised the hostel area, in case the sea level rises to an abnormal height. Before we built we advertised for a project manager and engaged Adrian Wakeling to live on site with his wife Coral during construction to monitor the project and manage the home because it had become a demanding task for the voluntary committee members. Adrian and Carol did a very good job and the clients loved them. They were a caring couple. They put in a lot of voluntary hours. George James' work with us had just about come to an end. One really cannot deny the great job these caring people have done for our people.

When we opened the doors to accept the clients, Rose Mabo was the first to be admitted. Dr Holt got back his sanity because the hospital acute beds were becoming vacant and the Rev. Fr Mullins' dream came to fruition, but it took us six years of hard slogging and we were grateful for the assistance Mura Kosker Sorority gave the committee.

The Torres Shire Council built the access road into the Star of the Sea Home grounds as a continuation of their road works when they were working around that area, and TRAWQ donated their CDEP workers to lay down the lawn we purchased from Cairns, and the community donated the plants which were also planted by the CDEP workers. CDEP means Community Development Employment Programs and the unemployed receives this benefit instead of unemployment benefits.

The committee decided to retain the name of the previous Catholic Aged Home and it was registered under the name of 'Star of the Sea' Home for the Aged. When the home began functioning George James suggested to me that the Committee should apply for funding for another four independent living units.

The committee requested George James to do the submission and it was successful. However, the new committee didn't allow him to continue to the end of the project. George then concentrated his work in Cairns and around the North Queensland area. Some of his Indigenous Work was the Yarrabah Home for the Aged and the WuChopperen Aboriginal Medical Centre in Cairns.

10

# Child abuse

In 1989 when Mura Kosker Sorority was first formed, Lena Passi discussed with me that the outer island women were very grieved about child abuse, so we approached John Scott from the Department of Aboriginal Affairs on TI for funding to bring some of the women in for a one day workshop to get their feeling on the child abuse.

John Scott approved and a cross section of women came in and the whole day was committed to discussion on child abuse. The agenda included:

- Main causes for sexual violence against children.
- What should they look for to know that it is happening?
- How should they respond and what to do when children tell them.
- What do they do with the offenders?
- How can they stop it from happening?

The outcome of the discussions was quite horrific. After the report, Lena Passi said that she was brought up in an environment where she was close to her uncles who cared for her and carried her without abuse. She and her male cousins had a good brother/sister relationship. She went on to say that, traditionally, we greet each other with body language. If we were to discourage physical contact, we needed to start some form of re-education.

The women decided that some form of education to the level of the children's understanding would assist to make them aware of the dangers and where assistance and support could be available. This educational vehicle indirectly was offered to Mura Kosker Sorority in the form of the Remote Area Aboriginal and Torres Strait Islanders Childcare Program or RAATSICCP.

The funding came from DFSA&IA under the Wayne Goss government, and Mura Kosker Sorority incorporated for their support for ongoing funding and co-ordination of the program. Mura Kosker Sorority during my time provided the opportunity for communities to focus on expansion of quality child care that is culturally appropriate. These programs were set up:

- The Aragun Child Care, Badu Island
- Poruma Kazil Child Care
- Darnley Island Child Care
- Dauan Island Child Care
- Nurapai Kazil Centre, Horn Island
- Arkai Ipikazil Kob, Kubin, Moa Island
- Weig Apei Kazil Child Care, St Paul's, Moa Island
- Warraber Island Child Care
- Kailag Ipkazil Child Care Centre.

The Child Care programs were run by traditional women. Mura Kosker Sorority empowered these women to take on the responsibilities, knowing we were only a phone call away if needed, but the Torres Strait women and their Childcare program developed their own identity and managed the challenge. I believed a lot more communities joined and established their childcare programs.

The Mura Kosker Sorority, under Jenny Vellis's Presidency, employed a staff level of:

Myself as the Co-ordinator
Lousie Ghee as the Administrator

Elaine Bin Juda as the Office Manager
Rhonda Doul and Maryann Gaffney as Domestic Violence Officers
Tony Gaffney as Domestic Violence Officer (Male)
Keith Fell as the HACC Co-ordinator
Marcellus Mills as the General Reliever
20 HACC Home Helpers positions.

Jenny took Elaine to the State Women's Conference at Yeppoon Resort, Rockhampton where I was one of the keynote speakers. When Jenny, Elaine and I arrived, we decided to get mileage out of the women's conference instead of whinging and bellyaching. So on the afternoon before I was to speak, the three of us discussed and planned our strategy.

Jenny was to speak first on the management committee role and the culturally appropriate strategy Mura Kosker Sorority has to consider, and the local protocol to be respected for an efficient women's organisation to function in the Torres Strait. Elaine followed with a talk about how to manage Torres Strait women in crises and how the Lena Passi Shelter is established because all this movement is not only new to the Torres Strait women but the men need to understand and be gradually re-educated to respect their women and the women to respect them too. That's why we have male employees.

Elaine and Jenny did very well speaking in front of 600 people.

During our lunch break, lots of people came over to our table to congratulate us on our talk. My talk was on women's issues, as previously mentioned throughout this book, and from experience I had gained attending the Women's Conference in Nairobi, Africa in 1985, as well as when the South Pacific Women assisted Mura Kosker Sorority and sent me to Geneva to the United Nations Convention for the Indigenous Working Party of the world.

11

# Geneva

Mura Kosker Sorority and IINA Torres Strait Islander women's group in Brisbane worked jointly preparing the paper I was to present. The only problem was the paper had 42 pages, and I only had ten minutes to present it. In Geneva the evening before my presentation, I had to start summarising the paper and, with the help of another woman living in the same place, summarised and typed as we went. We finished at 3 a.m.

The contents of the summary paper covered:

- Recognition of Indigenous Inherency
- Queensland Fisheries and Fauna Conservation
- Education
- Health
- Employment
- Traditional Adoption
- Human Rights and Equal Opportunities
- Politics
- Conservation.

I introduced my presentation by saying:

> Eminent Members of this United Nations Convention, Madam Chair, Ladies & Gentlemen, I give thanks on behalf of the

Torres Strait Islanders women and their loved one for the opportunity to address this Conference.

I will speak about the issues that are inherently Torres Strait, whether they be of our people in the Torres Strait or of those of our people who choose to live on the mainland of Australia.

My speech to you is a:

- Statement of Principles
- Statement of Concerns
- Statement of Being.

Of Torres Strait Islander women and their loved ones, I will begin with Recognition of Indigenous Inherency.

I found great difficulty in summarising 200 years of our life into ten minutes. Madam Dais, Chair of the Convention, smiled and said that I had almost used up ten minutes already.

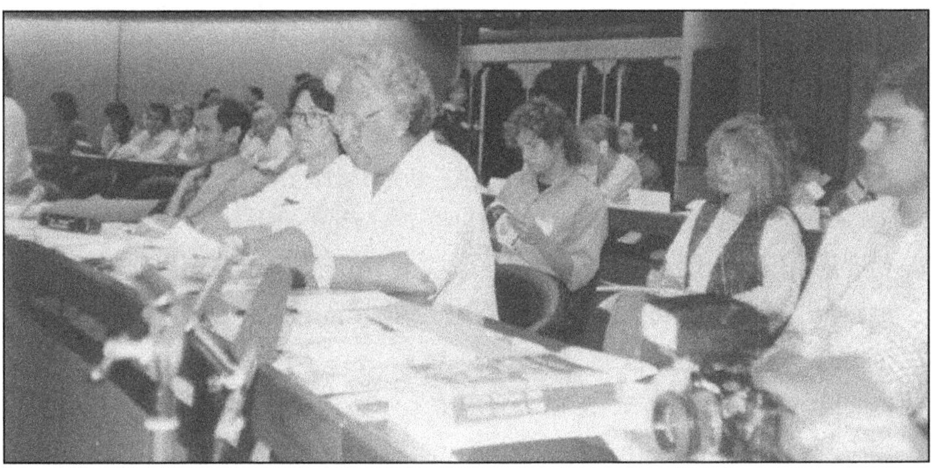

*Ellie Gaffney presenting the TSI Women's Paper to the United Nations Indigenous Working Party Conference in Geneva*

I was the first Torres Strait Islander to attend this forum in Geneva. George Mye followed and others after him. I commenced with our summarised version:

The combined Mura Kosker Sorority and IINA paper, the Torres Strait Islanders Women Group requests leave to submit into this 1989 Conference, the recommendations that were reached in concord after the historical inaugural International Indigenous Women's Conference held in Adelaide, Australia from the 9th to the 12th of July 1989 inclusive.

This forum provided the Torres Strait Islander women opportunity to establish a platform on the National and International level to project their views and concerns and make decisions and recommendation for improvement of their lives.

## RECOGNITION OF INDIGENOUS HERITAGE

For many years Australia has projected the image of a country tolerant of its Indigenous race of people which people were named 'Aborigine' by the establishment of the time through its Sciences Branch. You may remember earlier where I wrote that in the beginning we were under the Portfolio of the Minister for 'Flora, Fauna, Fisheries & Aborigines' in that order until the 1967 Referendum to remove two clauses from the Australian Constitution that changed the lives of the Aboriginal and Torres Strait Islander people forever.

Previously we were under the control of the British Commonwealth through the London Missionary Society to the governing control of the Queensland State Government.

It was from this annexure to Queensland Australia that Australia properly came into territorial possession of another Indigenous racial class of people, these people being the Indigenous inhabitants of the islands group of people termed 'Aborigines'.

The islands group was named Torres Strait after Captain Louis Torres. In spite of the patient suffering of this proud race of people who are known as Torres Strait Islanders, and which through blood lineage from my Aka Dadu, my brothers, sister and myself and our families are proud to belong. We declare this day before this August Conference of United Nations that within the territories of Australia there exists not a second Indigenous racial group, but two Indigenous racial groups.

To this very day in 1989, the State and Federal Government continues to use the term 'Aborigine' in its generic service when addressing the two Indigenous racial groups. This is both misleading and incorrect, indicating the level of real care and concern displayed by the State and Federal Government to its people, despite being knowledgeable of the fact.

### *Recommendation*

Australia and its territories possess two Indigenous racial groups, Torres Strait Islanders being one of the two and Aborigines being the other. Torres Strait Islanders call for the unequivocal support of this fact from the United Nations, and request that each nation duly in receipt of, and in support of this statement, bring to the attention of the nation of Australia as it sees fit within the spirit of support.

The next day my attention was drawn to a message received from the then Prime Minister, Bob Hawke, that his government had taken our recommendation on board regarding separation of the names of the two Indigenous races, for example, government departments and organisations became Aboriginal and Torres Strait Islanders Affairs. The rest is history.

## QUEENSLAND FISHERIES & FAUNA CONSERVATION ACT

Our Torres Strait people have developed technology unrivalled in the world. Applying to their natural environment, these skills are harmonious with the migration of fish, the cycles of the food chain both on land and sea, and are compatible with the time needed for the replenishing of these resources.

These dynamic traditional methods practised for generations provided balance between food chains and have from time to time been disrupted by the methods employed in commercial fishing. If comparisons were to be made between the methods of commercial fishing and the traditional methods, the former would be seen to be the major factor in the depletion rate of foods that are an integral part of Torres Strait culture and custom.

The various net line fishing methods used by commercial fishermen have seriously disrupted the dynamic balance and depleted the food chain plied by Torres Strait Islanders, for example, this depletion has affected the proliferation of dugong and turtles to the extent that the Department of Primary Industries has, through its Fisheries Branch, declared these two mammals protected. The reason given for caused this Order in Council to become effective was the depletion of numbers of dugong and turtle through the food gathering of the Aboriginals and Torres Strait Islanders. Little credence was given to the possibility that this depletion may have been caused by the commercial fishing and their practices causing injury and drowning of these mammals.

In view of stock depletions the Queensland Government by Order in Council placed a restrictions ban and a protection order on certain species of sea creatures that are part of the Torres Strait staple diet.

Correspondences had been sent on numerous occasions to various State Government Ministers responsible for Fisheries over a period of nine years, but had received no reply, including the Queensland Premier M.J. Ahern MLA who was briefed on the subject of traditional customs and methods of catching dugong and turtle but gave little joy towards securing the rights practised by generations of Torres Strait Islanders.

This practice by our people for generations has been sacrificed on the commercial altar with little regard given to the casualties or to the stated policy of integration concerning the same.

### *Recommendation*

Torres Strait Islanders seek international recognition and support of the customary laws and traditional rights inherently theirs regarding traditional methods of food gathering from land and sea and request that this United Nations duly notify the Australian authorities to advise them of this recognition and support.

On my return to TI, I was invited by the Island Co-ordinating Council Chairman, Getano Lui Jnr, to attend their executive meeting that evening with the Minister for Primary Industries, Mr Kerin, to answer the comments and recommendations made in Geneva at the United Nations Conference by me. I attended and explained to Mr Kerin that the Torres Strait Islander people, in Torres Strait and down south, found his restrictions too harsh on our people whilst his departmental officers here have on their BBQ menu marinated turtle steaks and dugong satays.

I was informed after that meeting that, with ICC support, commercial fishing licenses were reduced and restrictions relaxed for our people. The mammals multiplied and we were allowed to send traditional seafood south to our families. I would like to think that the Mura Kosker Sorority and IINA women's paper in Geneva was responsible for this with support and clout from Getano Lui Jnr and Island Co-ordinating Council members.

## EDUCATION

Up till 1985 the Education Curriculum was set for the Torres Strait people by the Department of Aboriginal Affairs. The highest education level to be attained was Year 7.

At that time our people saw no value or priority to attain higher education because encouragement to succeed was never the example set by our custodian of education.

Education was then transferred to the Department of Education where Year 12 was able to be attained by our youth who so desired. However, the curriculum was alien to the culture of Torres Strait.

Students from the outer islands must travel to Thursday Island to receive this updated schooling.

The language in the curriculum did not include Torres Strait language but German, French, Japanese etc. were included. Likewise Torres Strait history was not included but that of other countries was.

*Recommendation*

That the international bodies of the United Nations through the avenues bring notification of receipt of this address to the Australian Governments and its Education Department, concerning the vital need to include the Torres Strait languages in the curriculum, including our history, culture and custom at Primary, Secondary and Tertiary levels.

And that recognition from Australian Authority be sought by the United Nations of the far reaching implications of our uneducated body of people, the Torres Strait Islanders, and that this condition is a form of genocide.

And that the United Nations seek a commitment from the Australian Government to observe that international convention exists within the United Nations which clearly defines the need to adequately and properly address the unique educational needs of Torres Strait Islanders.

## HEALTH

The greatest threat now facing Torres Strait Islanders is the increasing prevalence of Sexually Transmitted Diseases (STD) and the march of both forms of Hepatitis B diseases (bacterial and viral) throughout the Torres Strait region.

Of the Sexually Transmitted Disease occurrences now besieging humanity, the Torres Strait – once isolated by virtue of its geographical locality – is now bearing the full brunt of, for example:

- Gonorrhoea
- Syphilis
- Herpes Complex
- Human Papillae Virus
- Human Immune Deficiency Virus (AIDS)

These diseases and their individual strains are the result of almost nil Health Regulations enforced in the Torres Strait. They are not 'intra' diseases as may be supposed, but are 'inter' diseases brought in through:

- Migrations of Papuan New Guineans
- Migrations of Indonesians
- Transit of seamen, and
- Other travellers.

The lack of a working knowledge of health related issues, being the direct result of the standard of education and the lack thereof, contributes to the situation.

These racial barriers effectively prevent 'self help'. This, downstream, contributes to the loss of self-esteem and eventual slide into a 'diseased culture'.

*Recommendation*

That the United Nations duly notify the Australian authorities of receipt of this major concern, and that it urge these same authorities, through avenues available to it, to attend to the dire need of:

- immediately implementing health education programmes that are translated through suitable Torres Strait Islander personnel;
- establishing, and supporting recurrently, community Health organisations that are run by Torres Strait Islanders;
- assisting Torres Strait Islanders in the establishing of an adequate infrastructure that will define health regulations and also enforce them;
- providing such support as is necessary for the existence of a community based Health Education Communications network that spans the eighteen inhabited islands of the Torres Strait.

Government departments, catering in full or in part to Australia's Indigenous peoples, are not adequately addressing the employment issues faced by Torres Strait Islanders in the Torres Strait and, to a lesser extent, on mainland Australia.

For example, no Torres Strait Island person is employed by the South East Queensland Regional Branch of the Department of Aboriginal Affairs. Though placements have been made available to Torres Strait Islanders in major government departments, no support systems exist that can assist Torres Strait Islanders to take up the many resources needed to bridge the cultural barrier, perhaps not regarded as important by institution workers but wholly part of the Torres Strait viewpoint.

The Aboriginal Employment Program established by the Department of Aboriginal Affairs is not holistically appropriate for Torres Strait Islanders, as its charter makes no room for the development of positions for women executives in the Public or Private sector.

With the nation strengthened, the current status has ample room for the establishment and development of employment for Torres Strait Islanders in Torres Strait and on the mainland.

### *Recommendation*

That the United Nations duly notify Australian authorities of the receipt of the Statement of Concern, and that what avenue of influence can be exercised by that international body, under existing or impending International covenants, be so exercised within a spirit of support for the perpetuation of Indigenous survival of Torres Strait Islanders.

And that specific focus bear on:

- Vocational training for Torres Strait Islanders.
- Creation of an efficient delivery of employment services, manned by and slanted towards Torres Strait Islanders (TSI).
- Other training courses for Torres Strait Islanders that are run by Torres Strait Islanders.

Since this recommendation the wishes of the Torres Strait Islanders, through the support of our Aboriginal brothers and sisters have come a long way in employment in various types of work and/or career.

## TRADITIONAL ADOPTION

Adoption of Indigenous children within their racial group has been a customary practice amongst Indigenous peoples, especially Torres Strait Islanders.

### *Recommendation*

That the United Nations duly notify Australian authorities of their receipt of this Statement, specifically that:

- In accord with the Melbourne Conference, legitimisation of Traditional Adoption be recognised at the international level with Australia being signatory to each convention;
- And that commitment be made by Australian authorities towards ratification of such convention in the short term, after signing of the convention.

## HUMAN RIGHTS AND EQUAL OPPORTUNITIES

To this date there has been no recognition of Torres Strait customary laws by either State or Federal Governments, or even Local Government.

There have been further amendments and regulations by the government to the preservation of National Parks and Wildlife, interpreted by Torres Strait Islanders as being an affront.

We are a minority group, where decades of neglect of the Aboriginal Indigenous race has spilt over to the Torres Strait Islands Indigenous race.

Human rights and equal opportunities are recognised as being necessary by all Australians, whether Caucasian or Indigenous. However this recognition by Caucasians is a 'hands off' recognition, consistent with their general status and culture.

This is not to deride the standards that exist for Caucasians. It merely points out the need for Torres Strait Islanders to embrace the condition of Caucasian people, to emphasise our Human Rights and Equal Opportunities, entirely without prejudice.

## *Recommendation*

That the United Nations duly notify the Australian authorities of receipt of this Statement of Concern, that:

- Torres Strait Islanders be given all assistance to access what rights are accorded them as Australian citizens.
- That these rights be defined specifically to meet the unique needs faced by Torres Strait Islanders.
- That the Australian authorities defining these rights conduct full negotiations with Torres Strait Islanders towards the resolution of definition.
- That Torres Strait Islanders be accorded the right to all of the resources available to Australian citizens and they are available across the broad social spectrum of the Torres Strait Islander community.

Torres Strait Islanders are becoming more and more sophisticated in their politics and the application of those politics. The move for sovereignty has been high on the agenda for Torres Strait Islanders who are despaired by the constant delay tactics of political instrumentalities.

At this time, whatever rights Torres Strait Islanders under Community Services Legislation enjoy, they do not allow for the principles of self-management and economic development.

The Kalamo Wacando case taken to the Australian High Court was rejected as Torres Strait Islander Independence was regarded as too much of a hot potato. At this time, the Eddie Mabo case for Land Rights is currently being viewed. Details cannot be committed to paper as it is still in the legal process.

Torres Strait Islanders have the right to practise politics in the local, national and international arena as they deem fit and know best. It has been observed that the basic fundamentals of the Westminster Democratic Political System are not unlike the basic traditional laws practiced by Torres Strait Islanders in their society.

Further, that the Local Government Act, superseded by Community Services Legislation, when viewed fundamentally, is a duplication of the social traditional system of the Torres Strait. There is no reason why the Torres Strait cannot have a Lord Mayor. Aldermanic functions and Councillors and Ambassadorial functions are also an inalienable right of Torres Strait Islanders.

### *Recommendation*

- That the United Nations duly notify Australian authorities of the Torres Strait Islands inalienable rights to practice political systems as deemed fit by them;

- And that the United Nations pursue international covenants on behalf of the Indigenous group 'Torres Strait Islanders' for the purpose of securing their inalienable right of political freedom.

Lots of changes and movement have taken place because of people pressure.

Today the Torres Strait is separated from ATSIC (Aboriginal and Torres Strait Islanders Commission) which is the peak Indigenous body in Australia, and we have our TSRA (Torres Strait Regional Authority), which was one of twelve grievances or requests read to the then Minister for Aboriginal Affairs, the Hon. Gerry Hand.

Also on the 3rd of June 1992, the High Court decision was handed down in the Eddie Koiki Mabo case, giving him and his Torres Strait Islanders their Native Title Rights.

At the present moment, ten years later, this is again in dispute with the Queensland Government and a land summit was held here on Thursday Island on the 17th and 18th of September 2003. I believe the outcome on the rights to the land for traditional owners was disappointing.

The Torres Shire now has its own Mayor. The first person was non-Indigenous, on a part time basis, elected in 1991–1994, not as a Mayor but as a Chairperson. The current person is an Indigenous person elected in 1994 on a full time basis as the Mayor.

The restrictions and delay tactics have virtually gone or are relaxed. Our people are eligible to run for various political positions because of the right of political freedom.

## CONSERVATION

The Torres Strait Islands being a volcanic outcrop of land in the South Pacific Region shares the worldwide concern over the Greenhouse effect which has gripped all nations, fearing the ecological disasters that will effect human and primary resources.

The Torres Strait Islands are limited to what they can do in this global situation but recognise and support the right to act on behalf of island communities. We believe that other nations can accord to what territorial actions Torres Strait Islanders deem necessary to invoke.

*Recommendation*

- That the United Nations accept what support and assistance Torres Strait Islanders choose to so enact, with existing and impending International covenants, and that such support and assistance be reciprocated when Torres Strait needs are imminent.
- In this regard strict control be established and maintained upon national commercial fisheries, in order that traditional foods (e.g. dugong, turtle) are not depleted from the Torres Strait staple diet.
- That International Conventions embrace the preservation of Torres Strait land/sea resources.
- That illegal entry into Torres Strait territories be monitored, and that prescribed penalties be enforced with appropriate actions.
- And that the United Nations duly notify Australian authorities of its recognition and support of Torres Strait conservation concerns and the territories.

Today in the Torres Strait, the Department of Immigration and Multi Cultural and Indigenous Affairs is monitoring the Torres Strait and enforcing appropriate actions for any breaches or illegal entry. The Department employs 20 to 30 mobile Indigenous Monitoring Officers and each island has two officers monitoring the traditional visitors movement under the Treaty. The Torres Strait office is on Thursday Island and, with staff of Indigenous blood lineage in the office and those monitoring the outer islands, altogether staffing is at 99 per cent.

## TORRES STRAIT TREATY

The Torres Strait Treaty is an agreement between two countries – Australia and Papua New Guinea.

This agreement was signed in December 1978 after talks, meetings and negotiation with the Queensland Government and the Islanders Community Council.

The agreement was to put a boundary line between the two countries and to advise which side of the boundary each one can travel, fish and use.

There are two main boundary lines:

1. The unbroken line is the Seabed Jurisdiction Line.
2. The broken line is the Fisheries Jurisdiction Line.

Australia is eligible to use the seabed south to the unbroken line and Papua New Guinea has the same kind of right north to that line.

There is a Protected Zone area that is special to the two countries. The main reason for the Protected Zone is so that the Torres Strait Islanders and coastal Papuans can have free movement and still live like before for visits and trading, with no need for a passport or visa.

The Treaty is set up for the two countries to work together to manage and share commercial fishing.

The Torres Strait Islanders can travel north to Papua New Guinea as far as to Daru (9th degree south latitude) and the coastal Papua New Guinea villagers can travel to Australia as far as number one reef (10 degrees, 30 minutes south latitude).

Traditional activities in the Treaty include gardening, collecting food, attending weddings and ceremonial and traditional trade. Visitors are not allowed to earn money or set up business. This is not traditional activity according to the Treaty.

The two countries have Liaison Officers who meet to talk, as well as the Fisheries Officers from the two countries.

The Quarantine law in the Treaty is very important and things

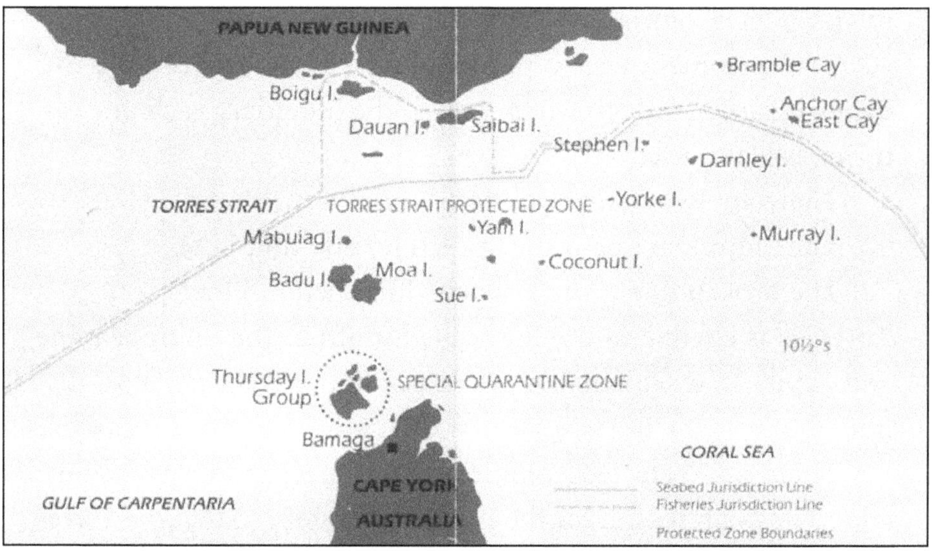


*Torres Strait Treaty zones*

*Source*: Department of Foreign Affairs, Thursday Island, brochure 'Torres Strait Treaty and-e you', July 1988

like live animals and birds, live plants, and fresh fruit and vegetables (e.g. banana, pineapple, Amniota, sweet potatoes and sugarcane) are not allowed into Australia. No meat from land animals or feathers or anything from animals or any eggs are allowed. These things mentioned are not allowed because they may carry pests and diseases into Torres Strait then onto Australia.

## CHILD WELFARE

The Torres Strait Islanders Women's group is most concerned about the necessary environment for the welfare of our children. Our greatest concern is that the cultural aspects of our daily lives must be preserved along community lines, through government sanctions and by international recognition.

### *Recommendation*

That the United Nations ensure that an International Convention be established for the purpose of ensuring that children be placed in a family of the same Indigenous racial group.

## DOMESTIC VIOLENCE

It is believed by Torres Strait Islander women that Domestic Violence is not as great a concern as may be experienced by other ethnic people. This is because the extended family group, in virtue of its breadth, contains inbuilt mechanisms that prevent the outbreak of uncontrolled domestic violence across the social strata.

This very same extended family group is the backbone of Torres Strait culture. It nourishes, generates, maintains, enforces and heals as the need arises.

*Recommendation*
As society becomes more complex, the rights of women need to be addressed to such an extent that there is national and international co-operation on the 'common front', for the purposes of safeguarding the rights of all women regardless of place, colour or creed.

The United Nations is requested to recognise this need and that, should there not exist International Conventions to the effects of the above, International Conventions be formed that define this right.

The journey on which the Women of Torres Strait sent me to Geneva for the United Nations Indigenous Working Party Group would have to be a journey one only dreams about, to be selected by the Women

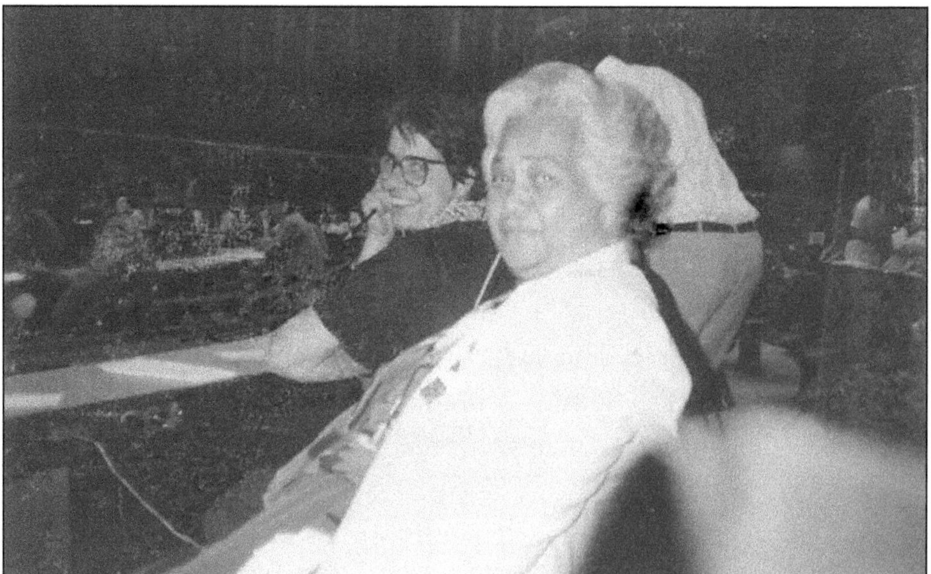

*Ellie Gaffney at the United Nations Working Party Group*

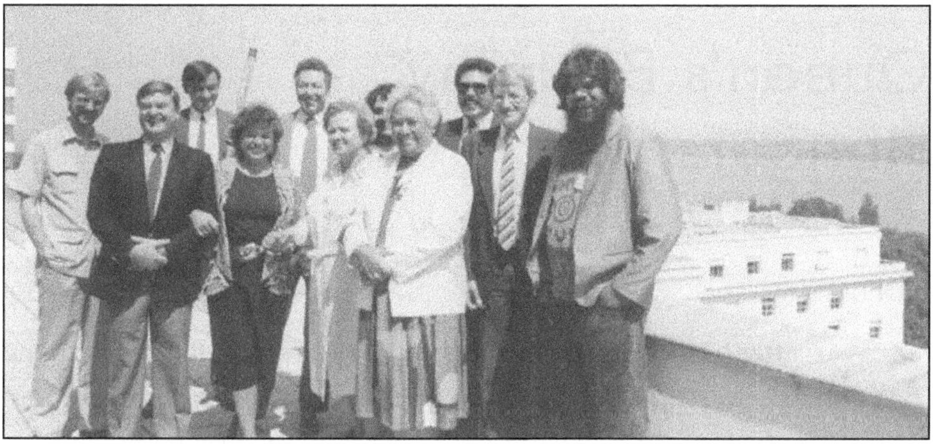

*Australian delegates with the Australian Ambassador and Madame Dias, Chair of the UN Indigenous Working Party Conference, at the Australian Embassy, Geneva*

of Torres Strait, on the mainland and from the Torres Strait. The journey was financed by the South Pacific Women and I was as a messenger for these women, to take their message to the platform of the world.

I am forever indebted to them for having the confidence in me and sincerely wish from the bottom of my heart that I have served you all well. God bless.

12

# Queen's Birthday Honours List

A year after returning from Geneva, I received a letter from the Official Secretary to the Governor-General, from Government House, Canberra ACT, advising me that my name was being considered for submission to Her Majesty the Queen for appointment as a member in the General Division of the Order of Australia (AM) in the Queen's Birthday Honours List.

I was advised that my citation would be for service in the community, in particular to the Aboriginal and Torres Strait Islander communities. Also he was directed by His Excellency the Governor-General to ask me whether I would accept this proposed honour.

Well, what could I say – naturally with all my heart and soul – 'I accept!' I received another letter advising me that the appointment as a member in the General Division of the Order of Australia had been approved by Her Majesty the Queen.

My insignia was presented to me at an Investiture held at Queensland Government House and gave me the entitlement to use the initials AM after my name as from the 21st of September 1990.

I received many congratulatory letters including one from the Minister Assisting the Prime Minister.

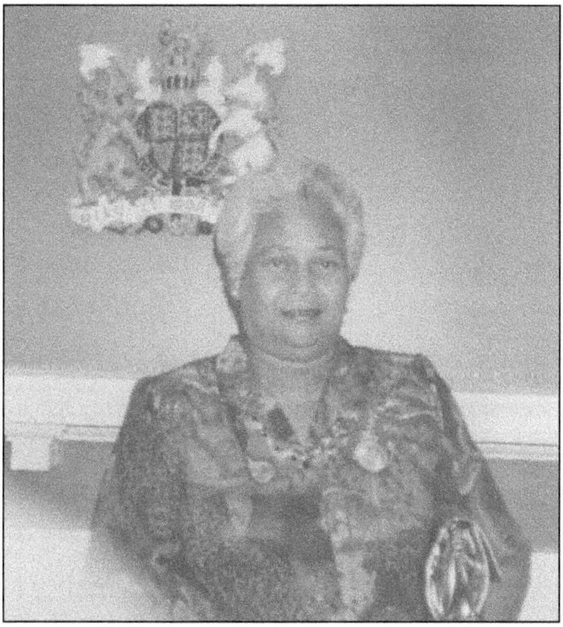

*Ellie Gaffney at Government House, Brisbane, proudly wearing her AM*

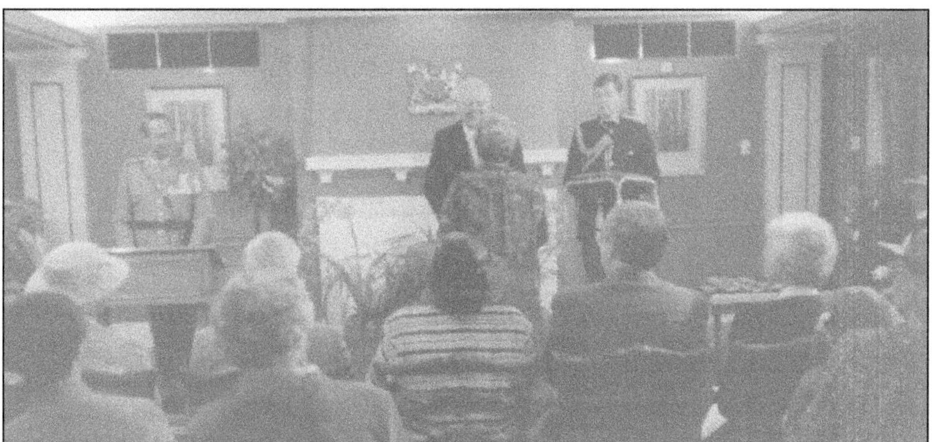

*Receiving my insignia*

## 13

# Mura Kosker Sorority, 1988 to 1995

From 1988 to 1995 it was a very busy period for the Mura Kosker Sorority organisation and the staff that I previously mentioned, with running the six services, and raising money to send women to conferences state, nationally and internationally. We sent women to Beijing, New Zealand, all around Australia – wherever there was a women's conference. Also the women did caravan tours throughout the Torres Strait to give support and encouragement to the women in the communities regarding the women's movement, which was something new and not culturally acceptable with Torres Strait culture, especially the men, at that time.

Our society's role for women was that we the women were:

- *Mothers*: to be a good wife and daughter in law by looking after the family with household chores, gardening and marital commitments; and
- *Daughters*: to accept one talk (delegation) from parents, brothers and older sisters for whatever is required.

On the hierarchal structure, the women were on the bottom in a servile position. They were not allowed to complain or have an opinion, and could be subjected to domestic violence for correctiveness by the in-laws (especially the mother-in-law) or husband. The husband had to slap his wife around if the mother in law was not happy with his wife.

No matter where you were in Torres Strait, if you were a woman, this was your life and Mura Kosker Sorority was about to change this by giving traditional women their human rights.

In the men's eyes, the women's voice really had no impact. However, because I had a track record of setting up legal services and broadcasting, as well as being a trained nurse who had nursed sick people and delivered babies, I was accepted by the menfolk virtually as their equal. And, having worked with Ted Loban and Joe McGinness, I was also respected and not categorised as a silly, stupid woman.

So gradually and respectfully, we sat with the community people and their Chairman explaining the movement and women's rights today and legal protection and services that are available, not just for women, but child care, education and training in any career the women choose to take.

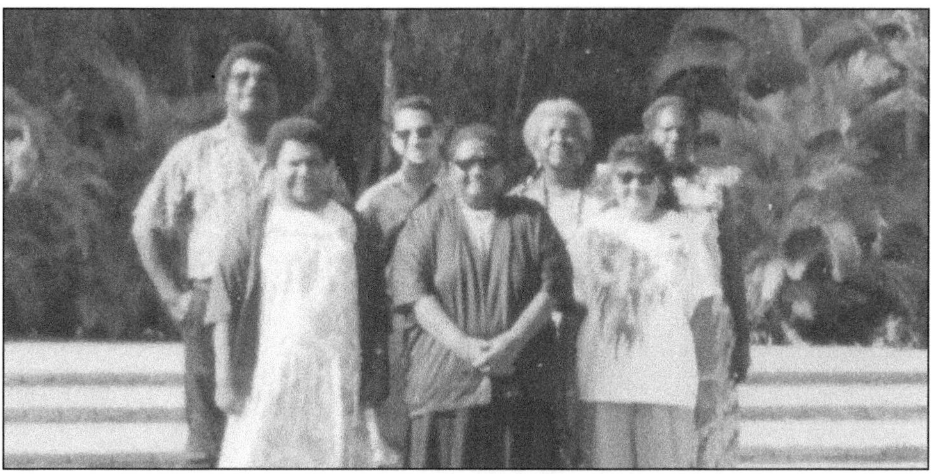

*The Mura Kosker team at the 'Turning the Tide' conference in Darwin. Front: R. Mosley, L. Ghee, Jenny Vellis. Back: K. Stephen, W. See Kee, E. Gaffney, S. Sam*

As previously mentioned, the period from 1988 to 1995 was a busy and highly industrious period for the staff and me. Besides establishing the Lena Passi Women's Shelter and the Star of the Sea Home for the Aged and attending conferences all over Australia and overseas, we supported Eddie 'Koiki' Mabo physically and financially when no one wanted to know him, except for John Scott from the Department of Aboriginal Affairs and John Abednego from our Legal Service.

Our office was well equipped with computer, photocopiers, faxes, electronic whiteboard, cars and lots and lots of money, and still ran effective and efficient services. It was the staff, and assistance from Jenny Vellis during the two years she was the President, and Val Schier working tirelessly and voluntarily during her time on the management committee, training the staff to be computer literate, that made it that way. As the Principal of the local TAFE, Val Schier led the women to

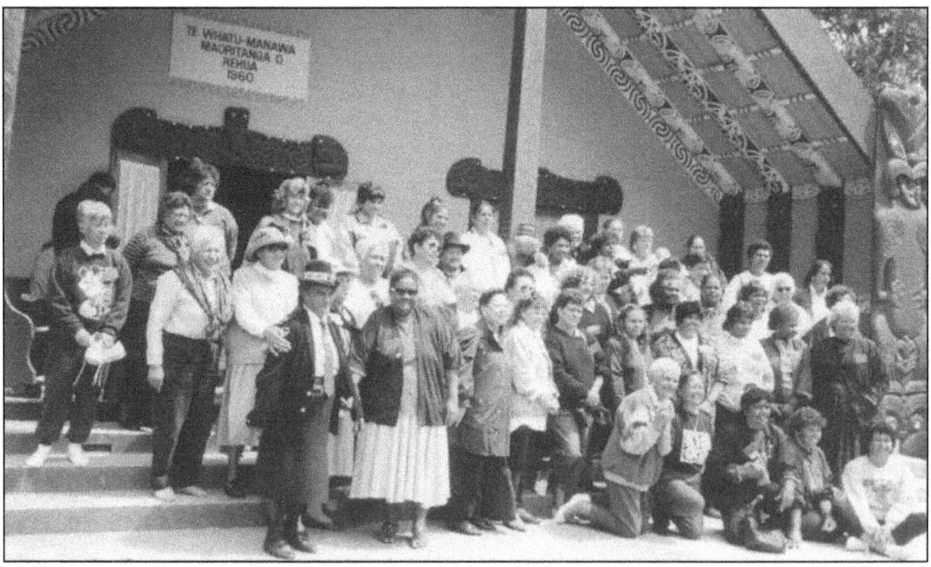


*Mura Kosker members with other international delegates at the International Women's Conference, Christchurch, New Zealand*

Christchurch New Zealand to an Indigenous International Women's Education Conference.

During our time in New Zealand, we visited their homes for the aged to enable us to check out their infrastructure and administration, as we always do in other places to give us ideas as to what was best for commissioning our Star of the Sea Home for the Aged.

Today, seven years after I left Mura Kosker Sorority, I am sad to say it has deteriorated, with no real services for the community. The services were discontinued or disposed of because of lack of skills to manage them.

I attended their Annual General Meeting on the 27th of November 2002 because of comments from the Minutes of the previous AGM and a suggestion to change the name.

The funding body, TSRA (Torres Strait Regional Authority) has

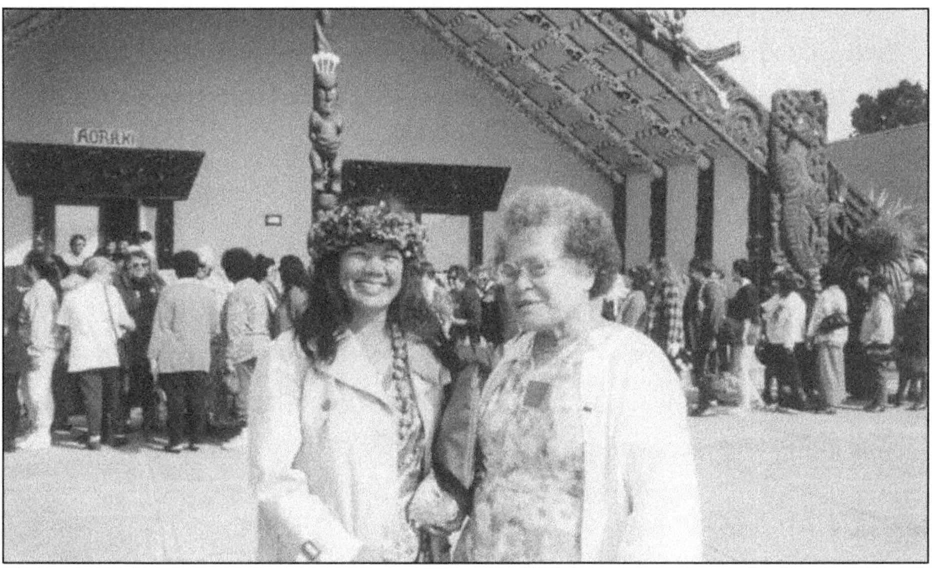

*Flo Kennedy with an Hawaiian delegate at the New Zealand women's conference*

questioned why the organisation should be funded at such a high level and recommended funds for only another six months, and to give a progress report.

The following are comments from the last three TSRA Financial Reports on Mura Kosker Sorority:

*1999 to 2000*

The Torres Strait Regional Authority funded the Mura Kosker Sorority $132,265. This was two and half times more than in our time but TSRA quoted their performance was ordinary as the organisation was still beset by administrative difficulties stemming from insufficient administrative funds to cater for various programs by the organisation. (This is not totally true because we had run these services without deficit. The real problem was that staff were highly paid for the job for which they were not qualified or experienced to manage, and outcomes depended heavily on the quality of their administration, based on honesty and integrity.)

*2000 to 2001*

This year's grant was $144,209. The Mura Kosker's performance has deteriorated further as the organisation is still beset by administrative difficulties. The other services were blamed but again I believe it was the highly paid staff who lacked administrative skills and experience.

*2001 to 2002*

Again Mura Kosker was funded $133,766 with no real services from the staff that they employed. TSRA now found the organ-

> isation was in grave difficulties stemming from an inability to organise efficient administration and that it was currently in breach of Grant conditions. The TSRA Board made the decision to closely monitor the operations and to limit their 2002–2003 funding to six months, at the end of which the situation would be reviewed by TSRA Administration.

What a shame, what a dreadful shame that the Mura Kosker Sorority had come to this.

14

# Ill health befalls

Several months later, I was sent to Cairns Base Hospital to a surgeon to have some investigation on my renal functions. Afterwards, I was advised to have an operation and perhaps to have a right nephrectomy, removal of the right kidney. After the operation, in the recovery room, the Surgeon came and saw me and advised me that the kidney was a healthy one and he didn't remove it, but removed a renal cyst.

I had moved to Cairns by this time, and just as well, because I developed complications post operatively. The wound was infected with septicaemia and broke down completely and was cared and dressed by the Community Health registered nurses every day, twice a day in the beginning, for six weeks, then daily for another six weeks. During this period, it aggravated my Diabetes which I previously had under control for seventeen years and I had to go on insulin injections twice a day. I developed Cardiac problems which resulted in other complications such as pulmonary hypertension, and spinal stenosis of three lumber vertebras, limiting my mobility.

The Cardiac specialist recommended surgery which I declined because by now I had had enough of invasive procedures.

I started back at work for the Torres Strait District Health in the Primary Health Care Section that was still under development. It was my 65th Birthday. I worked for three years to meet my financial needs and the District Manager, I believe, needed all the experienced and qualified Indigenous people available to implement his programs in empowering the people and educating them to take control of their illness or prevent illness for a better quality of life by different facets, such as eating more fruit and vegetables, no fried or fatty food, drinking more water, cut down on salt and so on.

Dr Elekana Faafoi was the overall Director for Primary Health Care but my Line Manager was Poyana Pensio, the Manager of the Public Health Unit. Poyana originally was employed with Queensland Railways. His responsibility there was managing people and programs and his work involved time, place and track and he managed the human and material resources to ensure outcomes were achieved. It was easier than managing the human aspects of health so he has been known to say.

When Poyana and his family moved back to the Torres Strait, he accepted the offer of the District Manager, Phillip Mills, to join him in establishing the integrated health services in the Torres Strait. Both Phillip and Poyana are the first Torres Strait Islanders to ever become Health Managers and Phillip was good for Poyana and must certainly have played an influential part in Poyana's life.

Together with the Chairperson of the District Council, Grace Fischer, and Dr Elekana Faafoi, with hand picked staff, the baby Primary Health Care was born and history was created.

We moved into the Primary Health Care Centre, 'SIBUWANI NURAPAI META', meaning the House of Caring and Sharing, on Douglas Street in late November 1997 and fragmented community health services became integrated. They continue to thrive even though Dr Elekana left us in 1999. Poyana applied for and was successful to become the first Torres Strait Indigenous Director of Primary Health Care for the District of Torres Strait and Northern Peninsula

Area. I was made the acting Health Centre Manager for six months to help establish and commission the Centre.

Two and a half years later we were still commissioning.

The Centre should have been commissioned before the staff moved in to deliver health services, but this is the result of a delegation coming from Brisbane and players with no health experience, especially in Health Administration. Phillip and Poy are qualified and experienced in health administration but the delegation came from the higher echelon. It took a long time to establish and commission the Health Centre, but the services continued efficiently without any interference. Credit and congratulations to those staff who proudly and effectively set up their units.

# Women's mental health

It is almost six years since the Primary Health Care Centre, the 'SIBUWANI NGURPAI META', was established in Douglas Street delivering Primary Health Care services – the Torres Strait model to the Torres Strait and Northern Peninsula Area Health Service District.

The model is the best I have ever come across, covering many different services, with Program Co-ordinators managing these programs and liaising with Cluster Co-ordinators for the four outer island groups, everyone implementing the Torres Strait model for Primary Health Care.

I am very proud of those Indigenous men and women who took the time out to get themselves educated in health and working with their Health Worker Services Manager assisting the Director of Primary Health Care.

These people assisted Phillip Mills, District Manager and Poyana Pensio, Director of Primary Health Care, to develop the Community Services with Health Promotion and Health Education, delivering the Disease Screening and Prevention Service with the Primary Health Care Services, and bridging the gap with Hospital based services.

Whilst I am a supporter of this model in Primary Health Care, I would like to point out that our women's Mental Health issues were never taken seriously because, I believe, once a women's issue affected her mentally, she was referred to a Mental Health Unit, which was predominately staffed by males and the only service for all mental health.

Before this happens, the woman should be screened to determine and identify the problem. It could be a mental issue from worrying about lack of accommodation, rental arrears, financial or whatever, then the focus should be accordingly appropriate, especially for any sexual harassment, rape or child molesting.

In 1988, the women recommended that a female Social Worker be shared by the hospital and women for women's business but this isn't happening. A female social worker, in my experience, is able to counsel both male and female, but a male social worker usually will have difficulty in counselling or attending women with issues affecting her mentally, especially women in the Torres Strait, from this multi-cultural race.

Here on Thursday Island, the women's bad lot has been increased with our fast-changing life, such as the many responsibilities given to women, not only wife and mother responsibilities, but securing accommodation, keeping the rent and other bills paid, ensuring there is money there, or going out to work because for various reasons the male partner may not be able to get a paying job.

If one goes out to work, they have to secure childcare for the children under school age. Only some of our men would share the responsibilities. In my father's and brother's time, they shared domestic chores and caring for the children as well as being the provider, but this isn't happening today, increasing the women's mental stress.

Very young women usually fall pregnant whilst at High School, or at that age because of lack of parental guidance, and these young females suffer from cross-cultural stress. They are advised to terminate the pregnancy which is culturally inappropriate, either through their spiritual belief or Indigenous culture. Should they decide to progress with the pregnancy and keep the baby, they are accepting a major responsibility and their youth has been robbed from them.

These women need intense counselling and direction in parenting skills. There are women's business organisations here as mentioned previously but this quality of service is beyond them because they lack the qualification, experience or commitment. Women's issues are not their priority to service. Likewise the District Health Primary Health.

I do hope that Primary Health will set up a special women's unit with a female social worker looking at all women's mental, physical, emotional and spiritual issues, staffed by qualified female staff, culturally appropriate, based on Thursday Island and with outreach staff. If we can produce a healthy mother mentally and physically, with spiritual belief, then we will have a woman that is emotionally stable which will produce a healthier family all round.

That is how I remember family life in the Torres Strait. Everyone was poor materially but rich with good health, mentally, emotionally, and spiritually. I had two religions in my life – my mother's, Anglican, and my father's, Muslim, and both teachings were excellent. Neither competed for favouritism, but both respectively produced a wonderful spiritual philosophy that has been the strength for our family's journey throughout our life.

And that would have been the case for other families here on Thursday Island, in mixed marriages with a multi-cultural basis that surrounded their family life. I can't remember any social mental problem, only psychiatric, retardation and that kind, at a minute level.

By early 2000, I discussed my deteriorating health with Poy and as much as I would like to continue working in health, I would have to be realistic and honest that I wouldn't be able to give 100 per cent to something I loved doing, and would be retiring. So in March 2000 I retired and the District Health through Phillip and Poy arranged a farewell luncheon with organisations and people I was associated with.

After retirement, I moved to Cairns again to be near the Diabetes Centre and Dr Clive Hadfield, the Medical Physician looking after me as my medical condition deteriorated and I was frequently admitted into the Cairns Base Hospital.

I found difficulty living on my own and had to rely on my daughters, nieces and grandson, especially relying on my older daughter, Whitney, and her son, Kevin, sleeping over, doing my shopping and taking me to the hospital anytime of the day or night. My husband had to stay on Thursday Island and look after our home and visited me in Cairns when leave and finance allowed it.

The crunch came when I was admitted again and the nurses were on strike. This threw the Accident and Emergency Ward and hospital into chaos with the shortage of nurses and wards closed down, reducing beds. Some of us had to spend long hours in Accident and Emergency or, in some cases, stay put in the ambulance until ward beds were available. And when we were accepted in a ward, it may not be in the appropriate ward. During my last admission there, I was transferred into three different wards in four days and was discharged before I was ready to be sent home alone.

I contacted the Thursday Island District Manager and explained my situation and he was sympathetic and suggested I return home and be cared for at the Thursday Island Hospital. I was transferred back home with an escort. That was fifteen months ago.

During my time back home, I was a frequent admission. Eventually after seven months, my admission was every alternate week for a week in hospital. I became very depressed because there didn't appear to be any interest in my illness or feelings, and the nursing care was not nursing care as I was taught, including the ward management.

Finally during the last admission in March (2003) I decided I would go home, no matter what, because even though it was a known fact that I had low blood count and it fluctuated, no one took an interest to restore it to normal level and I lacked energy, mentally and physically. In addition, I was on Warfarin to thin my blood and that had to be monitored because if it wasn't within the level required I suffered from the effects of it being higher or lower. The shortness of breath wasn't overload of fluid every time but I was suffering from some form of airway obstruction. When I got home, I was very weak and having angina (chest pain) more often than before. I couldn't bathe myself, so my husband assisted sponging me by my bedside.

My psychological framework was to prepare myself to accept what was to come and I really wanted someone to be by my side comforting me mentally and to give spiritual counselling. The person that came to mind was a family member, a respected elder who also belongs to the same tribe. So I sent for her to come and see me which she did. This person is Flo Kennedy, a wonderful, serene, spiritual person to whom I related my grievances because I had confidence in Flo to do the final journey with me with dignity.

I was not prepared for what was to take place. Flo comforted me and I could feel her empathy. She prayed for me and gave me water she blessed, and I remembered then that she was given healing powers from her dad who is renowned throughout the Indigenous race for his powers and health.

I placed myself completely into Flo's hands because I just wanted relief and dignity. Flo went further and asked the priests from her religion, the Church of Latter Days Saints, known as Mormons, to give me their blessing. The two Mormon priests came to our place on a Tuesday evening, two days after I came home from hospital. They explained about the blessing and proceeded with the blessing and oil application. That was six months ago and I haven't been back to the hospital for admission.

Flo spent the first month intensely caring and sharing her love and I gradually regained some quality of life. On visits to the Health Centre I explained to the two doctors who had taken me on as their responsibility.

They observed that changes had taken place in me and did some changes themselves, like trying to restore my blood level with iron tablets to lift my HB count from 5 to 13 and, needless to say, this increased my energy and I was only on iron tablets for four weeks and am maintaining the level on appropriate diet. As for the back pain, the doctor prescribed medication which rid me of that. I use it if necessary. This too gave me relief and better mobility even though I still use the walker, but without excruciating pain.

The shortness of breath which was the major reason for me to go to hospital has been sorted out by various methods. For instance if it does not really respond to anginacal or fluid tablets, then it's not cardiac or overload of fluid, so I resolve to use other methods which have been effective.

The blessing I believe was a miracle and Flo Kennedy was sent to me to do that job because I am not a Mormon but I have always believed Mormons are good people. They live good and they're good to people spiritually, physically, socially and emotionally. In my opinion they are good examples of living and I am forever grateful to them for giving me this new lease of quality life to enable me to write this book and sit on the Review Committee for Health to review and make a contribution to the 1993 Torres Strait Health Strategy.

# Women's health: An ongoing issue

The Women's recommendations from the 1988 Women's Health meeting have done a lot for our women's health and the 1993 Torres Strait Health Strategy Report, which touched on 'Women's' Health, also stated:

> ... one of the major issues related to women's health is that of perinatal health. The stillbirth, neonatal mortality, perinatal and infant mortality rates for the Torres Strait Region are all more than double Queensland rates.

The goal from that workshop was to specifically address issues relating to women's health in the Torres Strait Region by various strategies.

The neonatal/perinatal and infant morality problems have been reduced and a Women's Health Unit was jointly formed with men's health in the one room, managed by Yoko Nakata, and her male and female staff are efficient. However it's been fifteen years since Lena Passi and Marjorie Wymarra raised the women's grievances for better women's services to be established, and ten years since the 1993 Torres Strait Health Strategy Report touching on the issue again.

Women's business is fragmented and not complete as requested by the women over the years. I honestly believe that we here in the Torres Strait have done our best in creating awareness of the problems and establishing services in a fragmented form, delivered all over the place because of lack of accommodation.

There should be a place to pull all the fragmented services into one unit, to take care of the Women's Business from cradle to grave. The building required would accommodate clinics for antenatal and postnatal, maternal and child welfare, Pap Smears, mammograms and other women's health business, in privacy and with comfort and confidentiality, with qualified and appropriate female staff. This includes mental issues, whether it be social or emotional, financial or whatever.

There must be appropriate counselling rooms for privacy, a user friendly place for women and children to be educated, cared for and developed to overcome obstacles.

I found the current clinic accommodation, through no fault of the clinicians, is exposed to the public. For example, sitting in a thoroughfare corridor, everyone knows you're having a mammogram; turn the corner to sit and everyone knows you're having a colposcopy, and likewise for a pap smear. Other places overseas and in Australia, they have a women's unit, even in Cairns. It's time the women of Torres Strait had theirs.

Having said all that, I hope the review committee for the 1993 Torres Strait Health Strategy will include in its recommendations this much-needed Women's Unit to service the women from cradle to grave, with appropriate qualified female staff.

At the time I am writing this book, the review committee has had two meetings and will hold another before a huge workshop in early 2004 and the Director of Primary Health Care, Poyana Pensio will be travelling the outer islands with a staff member from Women's Health to collect data for the review before the workshop in 2004. It will be very interesting to see after ten years, if the 1993 Torres Strait Health Strategy has been a success. If not, then we must bring it to the attention of the custodian of our welfare in Women's Business and Health.

17

# Afterword

In conclusion, I would like to reflect on the journey taken throughout this book.

Firstly, my thanks to the women for their encouragement for me to accept the challenge, especially from Sylvia Tabua and my daughters, Maryann and Whitney, for me to make an attempt.

The FCAATSIA (Federal Council for the Aboriginal and Torres Strait Islanders) referendum anniversary is still celebrated by the Ware family, keeping the memory of their dad, Elia Ware, alive. Elia was involved in the Referendum through the FCAATSI movement.

The Torres Strait Women's Association led by Marjorie Wymarra and Eve Finney merged into another organisation for women, the Mura Kosker Sorority, which became one of, if not the most, powerful and effective organisations in the Torres Strait of that time. Unfortunately without proactive, dedicated leaders it eventually crumbled and continued to deteriorate.

The women's health meeting in June 1988 brought the women of Torres Strait and Northern Peninsula Area together to hear their grievances and suggestions for services required, not just in women's health. These included sea transport carrying provisions with a freezer and cooler to preserve the goods to be installed in the IBIS stores. Many more needs were projected and other recommendations made.

Currently the 1993 Torres Strait Health Strategy is being reviewed and ironically I am co-ordinating another 'Women's Health' meeting on the 6th of November 2003 to review the women's views for this Torres Strait Health Strategy and to listen to the women again on Women's Health Business.

As mentioned throughout the book, health service in the Torres Strait has been dichotomized into acute and specialist services at the hospital, and prevention, education and outreach services from the Primary Health Care under Poyana Pensio, the Director of Primary Health Care, established initially by Dr Elekani Faafoi.

The District Manager, Phillip Mills, is still the Captain steering the ship. I might add that, when he jumped aboard initially, it was a leaking wreck with many holes to plug up and the unsteady rudder needed to be fixed and steadied on course.

Phillip had a partner in Peter Heath, the Director of Corporate Services, during the time of development of the services and structural

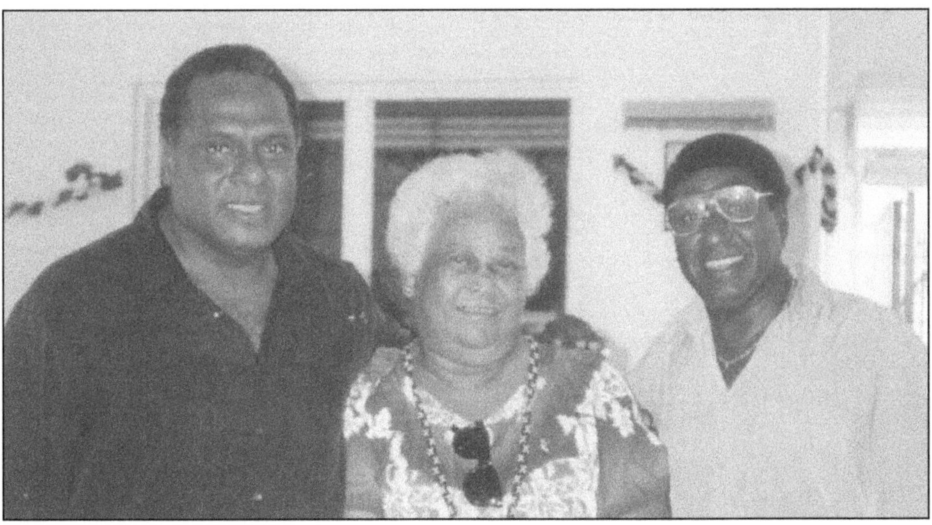

*Phillip Mills (District Manager), Ellie Gaffney and Poyana Pensio (Director, PHC) at Ellie's farewell lunch*

changes. I very much enjoyed working with him at that time, establishing the Health Centre.

The aged home is still functional but not the way we intended initially, but I suppose every management committee develops its own style of management. Our initial plan was to autonomise and Indigenously manage, similar to the Aboriginal Hostels and Yarrabah Aged Home.

I want to mention the love I have for the staff I worked with at Mura Kosker during the time we were all together, developing programs and implementing services, especially Louise Ghee. One cannot mention the women's movement without mentioning Louise – she was Mura Kosker and its success is a credit to her proactiveness, dedication, honesty and integrity and ability to administer and co-ordinate.

# Acknowledgements

To Elsie Ahmat, daughter of the late Joe McGinness for allowing me to include her father in my book.

To Phillip Mills, Poyana Pensio, Grace Fisher, Dr Peter Holt, and Yoko Nakata for allowing me to include them and the development history of health services in the Torres Strait.

To the Wymarra family for permission to mention their mother, the late Marjorie Gwendoline Wymarra, in my journey in reference to the women's movement.

Thank you George James, Architect, and Adrian Wakeling both for providing information and photos of the 'Star of the Sea Home for the Aged', and your precious loyalty to other people.

To the Kaurareg people for always having trust and confidence in any project our women put forth for their support, and approval to allow me to do things on their land for our people.

To the IINA Torres Strait Islander Women Group, the women of the Torres Strait and Northern Peninsula Area, together with the women from the Pacific group, for collectively producing material for the Geneva trip.

To Ann Marie Kirk from the Torres Strait Department of Immigration and Multi Cultural and Indigenous Affairs for assistance to me through the Torres Strait Treaty and update information on the Department's employment of Indigenous Monitoring Officers.

Finally to Charles Passi and Maria Tapim for photos and information on their late mother, Lena Passi – my relative, friend and partner in the women's movement.

# Appendix

## A National Aboriginal Health Strategy (1989), Ch. 7

Prepared by the NAHS Working Party, March 1989, AGPS, Canberra.



7.1 INTRODUCTION

This section is provided as a result of the Working Party recognising the distinct status of the people of the Torres Strait area. This section is written based upon traditional and cultural beliefs - which continue to this day. Specifically, these areas are shown in Map 1 below.

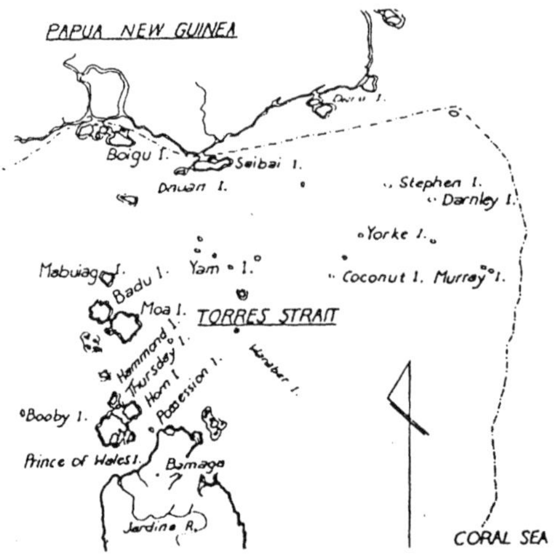


Map 1. The Torres Strait Region.
Source : Mr Billy Reid (Artist) in the Aboriginal Health Worker Journal (Volume 8 Number 1, 1984)

7.2 THE TORRES STRAITS ISLANDS

There are more than a hundred islands in the Torres Strait, of which fifteen islands are occupied and established as communities under a (State provided) Deed of Grant in Trust. Thursday Island was established as the administrative and commercial centre for the Torres Straits, whilst the Northern Peninsula Area was settled because of water shortages on some islands. Most of the islands are small, and many lack water which is suitable or fit for human consumption.

*A National Aboriginal Health Strategy (1989)*

*Source*: NAHS Working Party (March 1989), AGPS, Canberra, p. 115

The islands are usually described in four categories.

7.2.1 The eastern group :

This group consists of Darnley, Murray and Stephen Islands which are described as small, high volcanic islands with relatively fertile soil and dense vegetation. The total population is 684.

7.2.2 The central group :

This group consists of Yorke, Yam, Warraber (Sue) and Coconut Islands which are described as small vegetated sand cays built up on coral reefs. The total population is 708.

7.2.3 The western group :

This group consists of Badu Island, Mabuiag Island, Kubin and St Pauls on Moa Island, (all with a total population of 1,250); as well as the Port Kennedy area - Thursday, Horn, Hammond and Prince of Wales Islands (with a total population of 4,310) Each are described as large high islands, partly covered with moulds of basaltic rocks, lightly vegetated in open areas, and mostly well watered.

7.2.4 The top or far western group :

This group consists of Saibai, Dauan and Boigu Islands - plus those people from Papua New Guinea who may legally visit under the Border Agreement; and the numerous illegal immigrants. The population is 911.

7.3 SOCIAL HISTORY

The Torres Strait people have been lifeguards and protectors of the Torres Strait Islands since time immemorial. Torres Strait Islanders earnestly maintain their own identity, but are a caring and sharing people. Their language, legends, stories and other cultural activities are still practiced today.

The Torres Strait Islanders strive for equal opportunities and recognition of the rights of their indigenous heritage, as is the right of any sovereign people.

The importance granted to health is demonstrated by the fact that it was one of the twelve major grievances that brought together the Torres Strait Islander people in January, 1988 - during their attempt to secede.

The rationalisation and integration of health services in the Torres Straits is long overdue and is now a priority.

*A National Aboriginal Health Strategy (1989), cont'd*

*Source*: NAHS Working Party (March 1989), AGPS, Canberra, p. 116

While the Torres Strait Islands have been repeatedly exploited for their resources, very little has been done for the traditional owners in terms of alleviating basic problems in health, housing, food and other supplies, economic development and, until recently, education.

Because of the gross negligence by the State and Federal Governments of Australia, the Torres Strait Islanders fully supported the quest to secede. It was considered that independence was preferable to the abuse Islanders have had to endure. The British colonial law and order inflicted on the Islanders was never, and still is not, accepted by Torres Strait Islanders. Islanders recognise that as Australians, they have fought in the war to defend Australia. Underlying all the above, is the desire to be granted the basic human right of receiving a similiar quality of health facilities that other Australians accept as a norm.

7.4 CURRENT HEALTH SERVICES IN THE TORRES STRAIT ISLANDS

Health services in the Torres Straits and the Northern Peninsula Area are provided by the Queensland Government. The major problem has been that health services have been provided by different agencies - each with different philosophies and each with a different administration. Some have a limited degree of local participation, but certainly none offer community control.

The Queensland Department of Health provides the hospital services at Bamaga and on Thursday Island. Subject to financial constraints, clinics are also conducted on the outer islands. It also provides the Aboriginal Health Programme teams and the Maternal and Child Welfare clinic based on Thursday Island.

The Department of Community Services and Ethnic Affairs provides the Medical Aid Posts on each Torres Strait island community, the Maternal and Child Welfare clinic at Bamaga, as well as the pharmaceutical supplies to each Aid Post.

Current hospital health care services are neither appropriate nor effective for dealing with community health issues. The facility capable of managing a more meaningful and safe delivery of primary health care service would be a local community controlled health care board. The Board should be constituted as shown in Figure 2.

*A National Aboriginal Health Strategy (1989), cont'd*

*Source*: NAHS Working Party (March 1989), AGPS, Canberra, p. 117

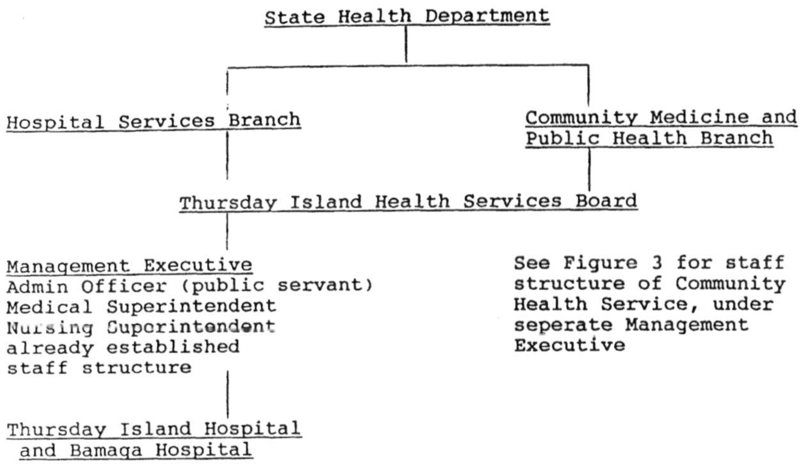


Figure 2. Thursday Island Health Services Board.

7.5 THE BOARD IN OVERVIEW

It is important to recognise that any rationalisation proposal must recognise the absolute necessity of seperating the Hospital Services from the Community Branch of the Board's Health Services. To help confirm and maintain this goal, both service branches will work for the same board locally with mutual liaison, co-ordination and co-operation, but with seperate budgets, management executives and control.

This Health Services Board should have the same charter (under current legislation) as a normal Hospital Board with respect to its ability to provide a full range of both hospital and community health services. It is important to note that historically, most hospital boards presently choose not to exercise their option to enter the field of community health.

The members of this Health Services Board should be appointed by the Minister for Health, from a list of nominees recommended by the duly elected, Local Government bodies in the region, using this model :

*A National Aboriginal Health Strategy (1989), cont'd*

*Source*: NAHS Working Party (March 1989), AGPS, Canberra, p. 118

| Number of Seats Appointee | |
|---|---|
| 1 | an appropriately qualified, in the health or management fields, resident of the Torres Straits; |
| 2 | Island Co-Ordinating Council nominees; |
| 1 | Torres Shire Council nominee; |
| 1 | Tamwoy / Abednego Council nominee; |
| 2 | community controlled Aboriginal or Islander organisations in the Torres Straits nominees; |
| 2 | Northern Peninsula Area nominees. |

Local Government bodies would obviously need to specify, in detail, their requirements in the selection process of the Board Members nominees, from which the Minister for Health would appoint a panel. Applicants must have relevant experience or qualifications to effectively serve on the Board - people must not be appointed in token positions. Where applicants do not have the above qualifications, then training programmes must be provided in order to enable appointees to contribute for their full term on the Board.

7.5.1 Staffing issues

Figure 3 offers a detailed staffing proposal for the Community Health Branch of the Health Services Board. Training Torres Strait Islander people in the delivery of health care needs to be emphasised. Whilst there is a registered School of Nursing for enrolled nursing aides at Thursday Island hospital, Health Workers need to be trained and given similiar recognition and the granting of accredited qualifications. Also needed is a program to acquaint non-Islander staff with the culture of the people of the Torres Straits. This could be undertaken during an in-service orientation and be provide through the same school providing the Health Worker training.

It is recommended that:

- the present Hospital Boards be expanded to the maximum number of nine members and renamed and restructured as a Health Services Board for the region.

It is clear that the provision of additional resources is vital to the improvement to the quality of life and health of Torres Strait Islander people however, the restructuring proposed within this section is of equal importance. Without Torres Strait Islander people being empowered to fully participate in the health care system, the 'missionary days' will remain and so too will the current levels of poor health.

*A National Aboriginal Health Strategy (1989), cont'd*

*Source*: NAHS Working Party (March 1989), AGPS, Canberra, p. 119

7.6 SPECIFIC HEALTH ISSUES

These may be described in three main categories :

- degenerative/lifestyle related diseases;
- sexually transmitted diseases; and
- imported infectious diseases - including from Papua New Guinea during traditional visits.

7.6.1 Degenerative/lifestyle related diseases

Diabetes/hypertension

- the number of registered diabetics/hypertensive indigenous adults in 1978 was 229, whilst in 1987, this figure had risen to 670. In 1988 there was 40% of adults aged 45 to 60 years old who were registered as diabetics;

- children are now being developed into future diabetics by well meaning parents and relatives giving them soft drinks, sweets, refined and fast foods. This risk could be avoided by ensuring adequate availability of appropriate foods through the Island stores. Diabetic Islanders are dying because the appropriate foods are not available in adequate quantity in all communities. They are dying from insufficient and ineffective health education programs which explain their diseases;

- remedial lifestyle education and behaviour modification programs demand a suitable community health service, not simply a hospital to cure the diseased people who are a result of the absence of such services; and

- this disease deteriorates and becomes a problem when most of the traditional diet is blocked, through a variety of means, from the Islanders and replaced by inadequate, inappropriate, and nutritional value food in the 'western diet'.

*A National Aboriginal Health Strategy (1989), cont'd*

*Source*: NAHS Working Party (March 1989), AGPS, Canberra, p. 120

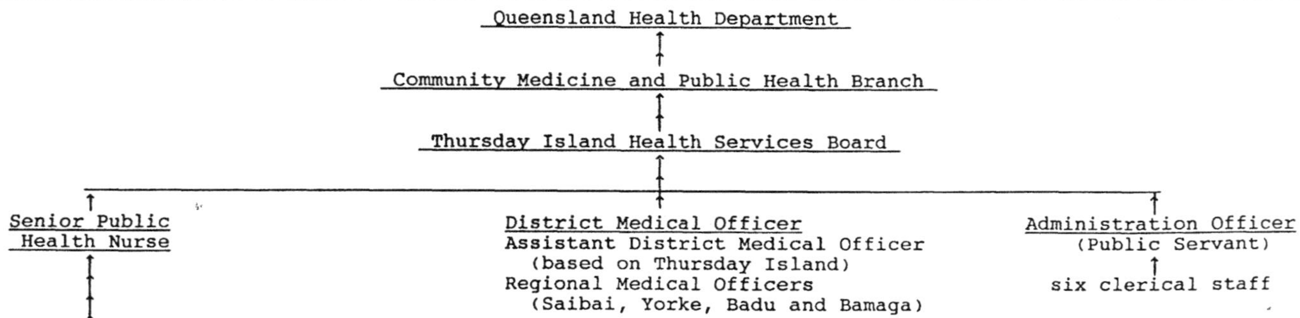


| Region | Public Health Nurses | Nurse Assistants | Health Assistants | Specialist Staff |
|---|---|---|---|---|
| - Bamaga | One | Four | Five | |
| - Thursday Island | One | Five | Six | |
| - Near West | One | Six | | |
| - Top West | One | Six | | |
| - Central | One | Six | | |
| - Eastern | One | Six | | |
| - Thursday Island | | | | Educator (Two) |
| - Thursday Island | | | | Maternal & Child Health Nurse (One) |
| - Thursday Island | | | | Diabetic clinic Nurse (One) |
| - Thursday Island | | | | Infectious Diseases Nurse (One) |
| - Thursday Island | | | | Relief Nurse (One) |

Figure 3. Detail of staff Structure of the Community Health Branch of the Health Services Board.

*A National Aboriginal Health Strategy (1989), cont'd*

*Source*: NAHS Working Party (March 1989), AGPS, Canberra, p. 121

The Working Party recommends that:

- an acceptable researcher dietitian/nutritionist be apponted undertake a detailed and specific study on the value of traditional foods in the Torres Strait Islands with a view to convincing health care providers, such as Governments, that the problem of diabetes in the Torres Strait Islands is serious.

Alcohol related

- a report was undertaken during 1988 on this issue, and evidence indicates a major problem exists. A community health centre on Thursday Island could assist health staff to manage alcohol problems, assisted by counsellors, social and youth workers. This would include visits to the outer islands. A community based health centre could also assist in the management of child abuse and neglect cases stemming from alcohol related problems in families.

7.6.2 Sexually transmitted diseases (STD)

Sexually transmitted diseases (specific)

- over the past decade, actual new infections of STD's from this region was approximately 3,300. This figure paints an alarming picture and has direct relevance to the following items.

Hepatitis B

- the prevalence of hepatitis B markers in the Torres Strait Islander population lies between 20 - 60% (depending on the community surveyed) with an 'infectious carrier status' prevalence of 29% overall. The hepatitis prevalence in the general population is around 0.2%.

AIDS

- the above situation for sexually transmitted diseases is of serious concern when considering the potential risk the Torres Strait communities have with AIDS. There have already been cases of death in the Torres Strait communities.

- unless a major campaign of education for behavioural change is attempted by an effective community health care service, there will be a decimation of the Torres Strait Islander race.

*A National Aboriginal Health Strategy (1989), cont'd*

*Source*: NAHS Working Party (March 1989), AGPS, Canberra, p. 122

7.6.3 Diseases Imported Durinq Traditional Vistits

- under the Border Treaty Agreement, traditional visits between Papua New Guinea and the Torres Strait Islands became legally permissable. This policy has proved a political maze, as well as socially disruptive to the Torres Strait Islanders. The transient population movement across the 'open' border is in the vicinity of 4,000 plus annually - most of which are not documented visits and most vistors are unlikely to be vaccinated against disease.

Malaria

- there have been outbreaks of (local transmission) malaria on the islands and as far as Cape York. Such outbreaks are expensive in the control measures required - these include vector control, residual insecticide house-spraying, mass blood slide examination and mass drug administration.

- the last two outbreaks have been more difficult to manage, since the vector control measures previously used are now socially unacceptable, and have not been replaced with a viable alternative. Furthermore, the malaria involved now tends to be drug resistant cerebral malaria, which is more difficult to treat.

Tuberculosis

- between 1978-1987, fifty-two new cases of tuberculosis have been treated in the Torres Strait Islands. The prevalence is fourteen times the State average for Queensland. Twenty nine per cent of these patients have been coastal Papua New Guinea villagers - either permanently or temporarily resident in Torres Strait.

Hansens (leprosy) disease

- there have been thirteen new cases of leprosy diagnosed in Torres Strait, five of whom have been infections, five were in Primary School, and nine were new cases. The probable source of infection was traced to one infectious lepormatous person, originally from a coastal Papua New Guinean village. This infection rate is 76.7 times the Queensland State average.

*A National Aboriginal Health Strategy (1989), cont'd*

*Source*: NAHS Working Party (March 1989), AGPS, Canberra, p. 123

7.7 CURRENT SOCIAL AND ENVIRONMENTAL ISSUES

7.7.1 Food

Availability and accessability - traditionally, Torres Strait Islanders were mainly dependent upon the sea for their basic food supplies and the provision of freight for other food stuffs.

The cultivation of fruit and vegetables in island gardens has been restricted because of lack of water, and because much of the suitable land has been claimed for airstrips.

The hunting for high protein foods in the sea is somewhat retarded because prawn trawling nets uproot the seabed and catch more than just prawns. For example, baby dugong and other food sources are often lost to the community. For Islanders to return to these nutritional foods, they now need to fish even further from their respective islands - this then requires a far more expensive craft which is totally beyond Islanders' financial capacity.

Therefore, Islanders are now reduced to a heavy dependancy on supplies of food from south of Thursday Island. Air freight is impractical because many Islanders are dependent on social security payments for their cash income. Air freighting provisions can prove very expensive with a small cabbage on Murray Island costing around nine dollars.

People living in the Torres Straits need to be exceptionally skilled in home management. Also, there is a need to ensure that there is adequate holding capacity in the island stores to reasonably cover the period until the next shipment. This is especially necessary for freezer / cooler, diabetic, and pharmaceutical lines.

The Working Party recommends that:

- each Island Store is equipped with adequate refrigeration capacity and general storage to ensure sufficient food supply - both regular lines and of diabetic foods - to fully span the period between supply ships.

7.7.2 Housing

Housing throughout the Torres Strait Islands is a priority. However, even though it is a priority, the Working Party cautions against rushing into and accepting the quick but high cost option. These houses often prove to be unsuitable for both practical and social reasons. Applications for housing should be processed by a Torres Strait Islands Commission of Housing. Applicants should be assessed according to three factors:

*A National Aboriginal Health Strategy (1989), cont'd*

*Source*: NAHS Working Party (March 1989), AGPS, Canberra, p. 124

- the needy and the homeless;
- length of residency in the Torres Strait; and
- traditional ties to the Torres Straits.

The Torres Strait Islands Commission of Housing should be formed by the amalgamation of all housing authorities in the Torres Strait Islands, currently between fifteen and twenty agencies. Not only would this reduce administrative costs, but community control and participation in the management board should reduce any opportunity for cronyism or nepotism in the allocation of employment and housing.

7.7.3 Water Supply

Although the Federal Government has funded water supply services for every island, at a cost in the millions of dollars, and these services are now at the stage of completion, the community consultation process found that nearly all the islands suffered some form of difficulty with water supply. On some islands, the water was visibly unfit for human consumption. There needs to be defined services to monitor the water supply and to train service maintenance staff - preferable local Islanders.

7.7.4 Waste Disposal

Because of inadequate waste disposal services, excreta and garbage is often washed back onto the beaches which then pose a serious health hazard. In some instances the people, mainly children, are walking, playing and swimming among faecal excreta. Further, the garbage breeds flies and mosquitoes.

Two qualified, health inspectors are required (resident in the Torres Straits) to service the Northern Peninsula Area and the outer Torres Strait Islands.

These staff would be to assist the Island people by advising appropriate sanitary/hygenic means for the disposal of refuse.

The Working Party recommends that:

- that, where no such system exists, appropriate waste disposal systems be planned and installed on each inhabited island, as well as in each of the Northern Peninsula Area communities.

*A National Aboriginal Health Strategy (1989), cont'd*

*Source*: NAHS Working Party (March 1989), AGPS, Canberra, p. 125

7.7.5 Access to Communication

Communication mediums in each community have been improved to some extent, however communication at the health care clinics needs to be upgraded by the provision of a twenty four hour telephone service. This facility is required for emergencies and to allow health workers to liaise with other health workers either at Thursday Island or at other clinics.

The Working Party recommends that:

- all health care clinics be provided with a 24 hour telephone service.

7.7.6 Power

The provision of universal twenty four hour electricity supply is not an immediate goal for the people in the Torres Strait Islands. Whilst it is desirable, it is simply not the most pressing problem today. It is hoped that this issue is considered and acted upon at the appropriate time and not simply used as a political issue.

7.8 A COMMUNITY DEVELOPMENT STRATEGY

Returning briefly to the introduction to this section, 'the rationalisation and integration of the primary health care services is long overdue and should be a priority'.

The underlying principle to the following strategy is that the community is given control of all its government funded health services by expanding the present Hospitals Boards to the maximum number of nine members and renaming it as a 'Health Services Board' for the region. This Health Services Board should then be funded to provide health services under two seperate branches:

- a Hospitals Section - operating the Thursday Island and Bamaga hospitals. The Thursday Island hospital requires upgrading of staffing and facilities to cope with the increasing population, and the full range of tropical and exotic diseases;
- a Community Section - operating a new Community Health Service which should be formed by full amalgamation of the existing Department of Community Services and Ethnic Affairs, Aboriginal Health Program, and Thursday Island Hospital Community Health Services. Because of the population, distances and transport availability to receive safe health services, there should be five regional doctors in the Torres Strait Islands, resident, on:

*A National Aboriginal Health Strategy (1989), cont'd*

*Source*: NAHS Working Party (March 1989), AGPS, Canberra, p. 126

- Saibai to service the top western islands and the international visitors;
- Yorke to service the eastern and central islands as well as the Papuan visitors;
- Badu to service the near western islands;
- Bamaga to service the five communities (Cowal Creek, Umagico, Bamaga, New Mapoon, and Seisa) of the Northern Peninsula Area;
- Thursday Island to serve as an Assistant District Medical Officer.

Additionally, there should be a small hospital or a larger clinic with some holding beds where a doctor is resident. The clinics and accommodation on the communities should be upgraded to meet the needs of both the population and the staff - doctors and health workers.

*A National Aboriginal Health Strategy (1989), cont'd*

*Source*: NAHS Working Party (March 1989), AGPS, Canberra, p. 127

# Name index

For Product Safety Concerns and Information please contact our EU
representative GPSR@taylorandfrancis.com
Taylor & Francis Verlag GmbH, Kaufingerstraße 24, 80331 München, Germany

www.ingramcontent.com/pod-product-compliance
Ingram Content Group UK Ltd.
Pitfield, Milton Keynes, MK11 3LW, UK
UKHW022201190926
475702UK00003B/135
* 9 7 8 0 9 7 7 5 7 4 2 0 9 *